12 <u>00</u>

The
NEGLECTED
CAUSE
of
STROKE

A Monograph in

MODERN CONCEPTS OF RADIOLOGY, NUCLEAR MEDICINE, AND ULTRASOUND

Edited by

LEWIS E. ETTER, M.D.

Professor of Radiology
Western Psychiatric Institute
and Falk Clinic
Presbyterian-University Hospital
School of Medicine
University of Pittsburgh
Pittsburgh, Pennsylvania

The
NEGLECTED
CAUSE
of
STROKE

*Occlusion of the Smaller Intracranial Arteries
and Their Diagnosis by Cerebral Angiography*

By

B. ALBERT RING, M.D.
*Department of Radiology
Mary Fletcher Hospital
The University of Vermont
College of Medicine
Burlington, Vermont*

Illustrations by

Margaret M. Waddington, M.D.
*Attending Neurologist
Rutland Hospital
Rutland, Vermont*

WARREN H. GREEN, INC.
St. Louis, Missouri, U.S.A.

Published and Distributed by

WARREN H. GREEN, INC.
10 South Brentwood Boulevard
St. Louis, Missouri 63105, U.S.A.

© 1969 by WARREN H. GREEN, INC.

Library of Congress Catalog Card No. 68-55659

Printed in the United States of America
7 B   53

ACKNOWLEDGMENTS

Dr. Waddington's illustrations speak for themselves. She also did much of the basic work on this subject, supplied several illustrative cases, and made many helpful suggestions in the preparation of this book. Credit for photographing the illustrations goes to Mr. Frank Mallory, director, and Mr. Wing Woon of the U.V.M. Department of Medical Photography.

Acknowledgment should also be made to the following persons at the University of Vermont Medical College and the Medical Center Hospital of Vermont: the Medical Library staff (for locating and checking references); the Neurology and Neurosurgical staff, and particularly Dr. R. M. P. Donaghy (for access to clinical records and their interest in cerebrovascular disease); the Department of Pathology and the post mortem services of the Mary Fletcher and DeGoesbriand Units of the Medical Center (who made possible the basic angiographic-anatomical correlations); Mrs. Nadine Gero and others in our file rooms (who sorted cases for representative illustrations), and Mrs. Barbara Hawley and Mrs. Elsie Stone (for typing the manuscript); my colleagues in the Radiology Department, particularly Dr. R. J. Hunziker (for allowing additional time for this project by assuming many of my routine duties) and most of all, to Dr. A. Bradley Soule, who made the whole thing possible.

B. A. R.

CONTENTS

LIST OF ILLUSTRATIONS

**The
NEGLECTED
CAUSE
of
STROKE**

SECTION 1

HEMODYNAMICS AND ATHEROMA
FORMATION

By REDUCING THE complexities of vascular degeneration to the simplest possible terms, it may be assumed that occlusive vascular disease is due to atherosclerosis and that atherosclerosis is a degenerative process based on both physical and chemical factors. The chemical or metabolic processes involve the entire vascular tree but the mechanical ones depend a great deal on local anatomy. Throughout life, arteries are subjected to stress by the pulsating blood pressure and the intima continually exposed to the abrading effect of the moving fluid. When blood flows smoothly, the layers in contact with the vessel wall move slowly while there is a greater velocity at successively deeper levels as though the fluid were moving as a series of sheets rather than a homogenous medium—hence the term "laminar flow." Such flow produces very little trauma to the vessel wall but when this smooth, almost frictionless type of flow changes to one in which there is swirling, eddies and cross currents the arterial lining is constantly being beaten and abraded and responds by forming atheromata. This turbulent flow not only predisposes to atheroma formation but diminishes the effective forward pressure in a manner comparable to friction loss and, once having occurred, is likely to recur distally with only minor precipitating cause. The factors leading to turbulence in blood vessels may be summarized as a greatly increased flow rate, an irregular or roughened inner surface, and abrupt changes in direction or size of the lumen. There is a formula, solved for Reynolds number,

[3]

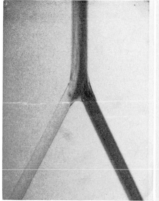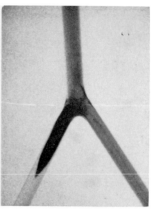

1.

LAMINAR AND TURBULENT FLOW IN GLASS MODELS SIMULATING
THE VERTEBROBASILAR SYSTEM. RECORDED ON 16 mm CINE FILM.

On the left, water is flowing through both arms of the vertebral portion
of the system and India ink injected on the right. There is a distinct linear
pattern of the ink particles with minor irregularities at the junction of the
two arms but no actual turbulence.

On the right, ink was injected as before but the left vertebral arm is
clamped and the enlargement made of a frame later in the sequence. There
is turbulence at the confluence of the two arms and ink particles are forced
back into the occluded segment in retrograde fashion and the ink particles
in the basilar arm are widely dispersed. The pointed end of the ink column
is similar to the appearance of the carotid at the bifurcation at angiography
when the actual occlusion is higher up in the carotid siphon.

that may be used to determine the probability of turbulence in linear
systems. This equates the speed of flow with vessel size, but is of
little value in the cerebral circulation since the flow rates in general
are well below the theoretical limits expected to cause turbulence. The
cerebral vessels, except for short distances, are anything but linear.
Of much greater importance is the configuration of vessels. Even
the rankest amateur home handyman/plumber knows that trouble
always arises at the bend of the pipe.

The earliest area of the vascular system to show degenerative
change, as evidenced by calcified atheroma, is the aortic knob where
there is a sharp angle in a vessel subjected to maximum blood flow.
The carotid sinus in the neck has two mechanical factors favoring
turbulence, the bifurcation itself and the slight bulbous enlargement
usually present. Enlargement of a vessel is fully as likely to produce
turbulence as narrowing. The vertebral arteries arise at nearly right

angles from the subclavians, an arrangement inviting turbulence at their origins. The left carotid comes off the aorta at right angles and would be expected to be subjected to greater stress than the right which comes off at a lesser angle from the innominate. The double curve of the carotid siphon would be expected to disturb smooth flow patterns, which it does, as shown by the frequency with which this location is the site of occlusions, being second only to the carotid bifurcation in the frequency of involvement.

The above areas are anatomical and exist in all individuals. Factors such as hypertension or diabetes would, of necessity, affect all these areas. From these simple facts, it is possible to draw two conclusions:

(1) Although it is known that severe stenosis or occlusions protect the vessels distally from degenerative change, this does not occur until the stenosis is sufficiently severe to reduce blood flow which is thought to occur only with a narrowing of over 50%. With less narrowing, the intracranial arteries are not only exposed to the same factors causing atheroma in the neck vessels but may be further damaged by the tendency of turbulence to recur after it has been exaggerated by the irregular plaques in the extracranial arteries. Consequently, **intracranial vascular degeneration would be expected to coexist with extracranial changes in many individuals.**

(2) Perhaps more important is the obvious point, that since the anatomical predispositions are multiple, a **multiplicity of lesions involving the extracranial vessels should be expected in older individuals** as a logical expression of vascular aging.

The significance of these atheromata is an entirely different matter. Doctor Eddy and I found calcified atheroma in the carotid sinus in the majority of patients over 70 and there seemed to be no connection between the atheromata as manifested by the visible calcification and evidence of clinical cerebrovascular disease. The pathology produced by atherosclerosis, as stated by Jett and Grundy, is not as much by its presence as by the speed of development and the significance can be better understood by applying the concept of Delarve and Gouygu, who divide the manifestations of atherosclerosis into primary and secondary. The primary effect is that of a mass in the vessel wall that, if large enough, may cause narrowing. The secondary effects of atherosclerosis are ulceration of an atheromatous plaque with thrombus formation and distal emboli, hemorrhage into a plaque which pushes it into the lumen and occludes the vessel, or evacuation of an ulcerated plaque with emboli of calcific debris and cholesterol crystals. Where primary atherosclerosis tends to be generalized and predictable following definite anatomical patterns, the secondary manifestations are accidental, not predictable, and occur under conditions that are not thoroughly understood. These are the early killers and cripplers and may be highly localized with only minor evidence of vascular degeneration elsewhere. It seems likely that much of the confusion in the entire picture of cerebrovascular disease has developed from a tendency to consider all manifestations of atherosclerosis in the same light. The slowly progressing, densely calcified atherosclerosis of the elderly has little more similarity to the acutely ulcerated thrombus covered plaque of the younger individual than scabies to leprosy and to consider the two processes as identical would seem no more logical than considering all acid fast bacilli in the urine as identical, whether they were Mycobacterium tuberculosi or M. smegmatis.

PROTECTIVE MECHANISM IN CEREBRAL CIRCULATION

From the preceding, it might appear that the extracranial vessels were sowing the seed of their own destruction in their anatomical peculiarities that invite degenerative change. The protective potentials of the brain's blood supply, however, compensate for stenoses and occlusion in an amazingly efficient manner. The best known of the compensating mechanisms is through the great anastamotic circle at the base of the brain described by Sir Thomas Willis in 1664 and the function of these anastomoses have been extensively discussed. All investigators since the pioneer work of Riggs in 1938 have found that a complete, well-developed circle of Willis is the exception rather than the rule. The individual components are not often absent but frequently are so tiny that no significant collateral is possible if a sudden occlusion occurs. It does appear that, if given time, as with a gradual stenosis, these small anastomotic channels may enlarge sufficiently to be useful.

In addition to the collaterals through the circle of Willis, there are abundant connections between internal and external carotid circulation, the most important being through the opthalmic artery from the internal facial. This was described by Elschnig in 1893 and demonstrated angiographically by Marx in 1949. Other common routes are through the meningeal vessels directly or less often through the "rete mirabile," or an additional supply to the vertebral artery by way of the occipital branch of the external carotid. Torkildsen and

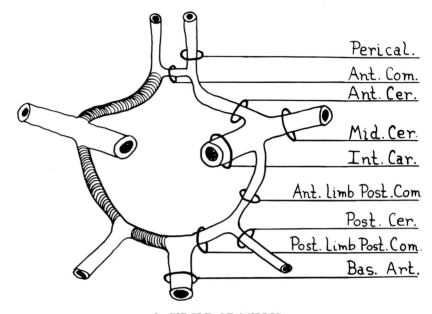

Perical.

Ant. Com.

Ant. Cer.

Mid. Cer.

Int. Car.

Ant. Limb Post.Com

Post. Cer.

Post. Limb Post.Com.

Bas. Art.

2. CIRCLE OF WILLIS

Schematic drawing of circle of Willis, the shading representing areas commonly deficient—not, obviously, all in the same patient or all on the same side.

The connection between carotid and basilar artery is made up of two components, that between basilar and posterior cerebral arteries and between posterior cerebral and carotid. When the posterior ramus of the posterior communicating is small or atretic, the posterior cerebral is functionally a branch of the carotid.

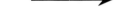

3. COLLATERAL CIRCULATION BETWEEN EXTERNAL AND INTERNAL CAROTID BRANCHES

Excellent collateral circulation through the ophthalmic artery with normal intracranial branches, also opacification of the basilar and posterior cerebral arteries from collateral between the occipital branch of the external carotid and the muscular branches of the vertebral. Such efficient collateral explains the asymptomatic internal carotid occlusions. Filling of the pericallosal groups is not the usual finding and in this case was due to a recent occlusion of the opposite carotid. The patient's difficulties were due to a large intracranial embolus on the side of the recent carotid occlusion. This condition is discussed subsequently under the heading of concealed emboli.

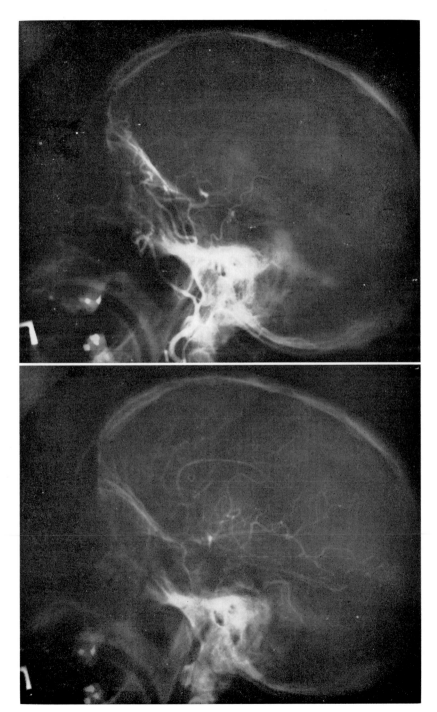

3. COLLATERAL CIRCULATION: 3A (*Upper*), 3B (*Lower*).
See legend, page 8.

the Norwegian group were early contributors to our knowledge of this collateral which may be so efficient that delayed films at carotid angiography sometimes show a perfectly normal intracerebral arterial pattern in the presence of complete occlusion of the internal carotid.

The vertebral arteries have segmental branches as opposed to the internal carotid. These anastomose freely with vessels present in the richly vascularized musculature of the neck allowing collateral circulation not only through the circle of Willis, in cases of carotid occlusion, but to the vertebral itself when this is occluded below the level of C1.

There is also anastomotic communication through the small pial vessels that are important in intracranial occlusions. There are a number of articles in the literature dealing with various aspects of

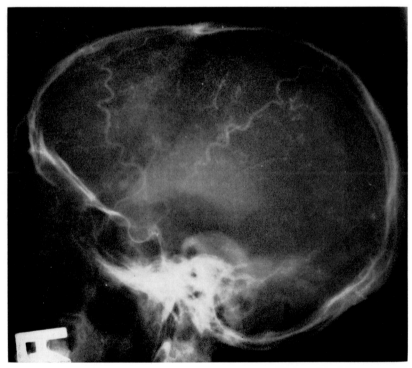

4. COLLATERAL CIRCULATION THROUGH THE "RETE MIRABILE"

This is a less common form of collateral between internal and external carotid branches, but gives a striking angiographic appearance simulating a meningioma.

cerebral collateral circulation and a comprehensive review may be found in the monograph by Fields and colleagues. More recently, the various collateral routes were summarized by Lee and Hodes, and Hawkins.

The arrangement of the vertebrobasilar axis is in itself a protective mechanism. The arrangement of two arteries fusing to form one is unique and allows the area to be supplied by either artery if one is compromised. Compression of one vertebral artery by bony spurs on turning the head is a current popular concept in the production of cerebrovascular disease. If this occurs, it should be compensated by increased flow in the opposite vertebral. In experimental studies, using glass models simulating the vertebrobasilar trunk and adjusting the resistance to deliver the approximate volume found in the human, we found total flow to be reduced by less than 10% when the tube leading to one of the vertebral arms of the system was clamped. Unfortunately, as in the circle of Willis, there are many anomalies that negate the potential usefulness of the system in some individuals. Unequal sized vertebral arteries are the rule rather than the exception and one, the right especially, is not infrequently so small that it has no functional connection with the basilar. The potentials for successful collateral circulation, then, vary with the anatomy of the individual concerned.

Although the above facts are very basic and important, like most good things they can be overdone. The possibility of explaining multiple manifestations of cerebrovascular disease by impaired collateral circulation due to anatomic variants has probably contributed appreciably to the emphasis placed on the great cerebral vessels in the neck to the exclusion of intracerebral factors.

HISTORICAL – DEVELOPMENT OF CURRENT CONCEPTS

THE ENTHUSIASMS FOR concepts relating cerebrovascular disease to occlusive processes of the great vessels in the neck may have its origin in part in the fortuitous coincidental development of cerebral angiography, reconstructive vascular surgery, anticoagulant therapy and the new theories that were ideal for the application of these techniques. Much of the basic pathology of cerebrovascular disease had been documented prior to the twentieth century and "spasm" as a cause of stroke was suggested by Peabody in 1891. However, there seemed to be little clinical interest in cerebrovascular disease apart from academicians and the clinical application at the turn of the century is probably well summarized in the cryptic notes of a late friend and benefactor, Dr. Edwin F. Pearce, who was a medical student at that time. On the margin of the section on cerebrovascular disease in his neurology text (Starr: *Diseases of the Nervous System*) is written "—9 out of 10 cases can't tell if it's hemorrhage, embolus or thrombosis." Similar statements with more authoritative bases were made half a century later (see references to Dalsgaard Nielsen and Bull). The curiosity of the medical mind kept research alive in this field despite clinical apathy although at a relatively slow pace. Chiari documented the clinical and pathological findings of internal carotid occlusion in 1905, but at the same time pointed out that the lesions at the bifurcation of the carotid gave rise to intracranial emboli. An earlier version of today's "transient ischemic attack" was the term "cerebral intermittent claudication" used by Hunt in 1914 in an article emphasizing the importance of the extracranial carotid arteries in cerebrovascular disease. Sporadic cases of carotid occlusions were reported subsequently but there were no large post mortem series until Hultquist in 1942 reported finding 91 cases of carotid artery occlusion from a large autopsy series. After a hiatus of several years, perhaps because of World War II, reports of a similar nature appeared including those by Fisher, Hutchinson and Yates, Samuels; Martin, Whisnant and Sayre, and Swartz and Mitchel.

Prior to and during the period that this information was being obtained, there was a general concern by neurologists and some neuropathologists over the frequency with which no anatomical explanation was found for cerebral vascular accidents. This was expressed in Aring's paper in 1945 where, noting the frequency of "negative" intracranial findings in cases of stroke, he stated — "since the physiological control of cerebral circulation is largely extracerebral, it logically follows that the blow that finally unbalances this marvelously steady mechanism must usually originate extracerebrally." The doctrine of spasm was revived, perhaps because at the moment there was nothing better and the human intellect, as well as nature, abhors a vacuum. The concept of extracerebral factors has never lost its appeal. Aring's work was reinforced by that of Wilson and colleagues in 1951 who stated, "what happens to the total cerebral blood flow in the last analysis depends on factors largely extracerebral." Gormsen and his group ten years later pointed out the frequency of cardiac disease associated with cerebral accidents and implicated reduced cardiac output as well as possible emboli. Chase and Kricheff, in 1966, discussing the radiology of cerebrovascular disease, mention extracerebral factors as possible explanations for the inconclusive angiograms in the presence of clinical stroke.

Although spasm as an entity was developed for want of a better explanation of some cases of cerebrovascular disease, its popularity died hard after a lingering decline.

This does not imply that spasm as such does not occur. The vasospastic phenomenon of migraine is in a category by itself. The secondary spasm that may pose serious problems in relation to aneurysms or other abnormal intracranial conditions or be produced by traumatizing a vessel is a very real entity that should be differentiated from the theoretical spasm that was assumed to arise de novo and persist long enough to produce cerebral infarction. Pickering raised objections to this theoretical spasm in 1948 and again in 1952, but its final demise—if it has occurred—is probably due to its replacement by another mechanism that was better suited for the times. This was introduced by Denny-Brown in 1951 and is so basic to the current concepts of occlusive cerebrovascular disease that it is worth quoting in some detail. A series of patients with similar symptoms and angiographic findings of carotid occlusion formed the basis for the report. After discounting "spasm" as being responsible for crises in cerebral hemodynamics, the question was asked, "What is the basis for repeated weakness of the left arm or repeated dysphasia, for example, with recovery in the interim?" "An answer to this question is, I believe, offered by cases of chronic occlusion of the internal carotid artery and similar occlusions of the basilar artery." The article continues that when either of these vessels were suddenly occluded, severe and rapidly-fatal coma usually resulted, but "more gradual chronic stenosis produces a state of episodic insufficiency in the circle of Willis which is responsible for recurrent attacks of paralytic phenomena." This work was received with enthusiasm. Corday and colleagues, in 1953, in describing the concept of cerebral vascular insufficiency as a "new" entity, referred to temporary cerebral dysfunction following thrombosis of the carotid artery as the "Denny-Brown syndrome."

Although Denny-Brown's work marked the beginning of the end of the concept of vascular spasm, it instituted the beginning of the cult of the great vessels. For the first time, theory and practice could be united and applied to treatment. On a theoretical plane, the new concept was grafted directly on existing theories of extracerebral factors in cerebrovascular disease and on a practical level the lesions could be diagnosed angiographically and were potentially curable by surgery. These concepts were given support in authoritative texts and after Eastcott, Pickering and Rob described the first successful carotid endarterectomy in 1954 enthusiasm knew no bounds. The field was new, stimulating and exciting, and there was an abundance of clinical material. Where but few could hope to duplicate the massive series of brain tumors accumulated by a Cushing or an Olivekrona, cerebrovascular disease, as one of the most common problems in the world, was so prevalent that the number of cases examined or treated were limited only by the staying power of the interested physician. The expanding use of carotid angiography was given further impetus by papers by Dalsgaard-Nielsen and Bull who reported the inadequacy of clinical diagnosis. From this time on, the literature is so voluminous that it is impossible to give credit to all who made advances in the field. In the radiological literature, there were so many reports that the editors of the *Year Book of Radiology* for 1959-60 noted angiographic investigation of carotid and cerebral atherosclerosis second in popularity only to the then pressing problem of hazards of ionizing radiation. The use of a catheter in the aorta to opacify all four cerebral vessels in their cervical portions at one examination, as suggested by Gensini and Ecker in 1961 tended, in many institutions, to move extracranial vascular lesions from the province of the neurosurgeon and neurologist to the vascular surgeon. When Seldinger's technique was generally applied to this procedure, and other avenues of approach besides the femoral vessels were available, four-vessel angiography became the sine qua non of the investigation of cerebrovascular disease. This procedure, in company with the term "transient ischemic attack," became the mainstay of the proponents of lesions of the extracranial arteries as the primary cause of cerebrovascular disease.

SECTION 4

SIGNIFICANCE OF EXTRACRANIAL STENOSES
AND OCCLUSIONS

IT IS DIFFICULT to assess the true significance of stenoses and occlusions of the neck vessels in the production of cerebrovascular disease for many reasons. One of the most important lies in the basic thoughts behind current popular concepts. This can be expressed in pseudo-mathematical fashion in a formula equating cerebrovascular disease with one known, the offending stenosis or occlusion, and several unknowns, the anatomy of the individual's collateral pathways and the efficiency of flow through them, plus the intracranial resistance and extracerebral factors. Such an equation, having more unknowns than knowns, is called indeterminate and can be considered either unsolvable or solved by assuming an infinite number of answers. (Judging from the number of reports in the literature, the latter course seems to have been preferred).

The "known" portion of the equation is improved by studying all four cerebral vessels since nonsymptom-producing stenoses of others may play a part in the production of disease by decreasing the total flow. The "aortic arch study," opacifying all four vessels at one examination, is certainly advantageous in picking up anatomical defects but does have the disadvantage of masking the hemodynamics of collateral around the circle of Willis that is sometimes striking when one vessel is studied at a time. However, no matter how complete the knowledge of the extracranial vessels, there are, except in extreme

[16]

cases, still more variables than knowns and the equation remains indeterminate.

The statistical approach may be applied to this problem by finding the incidence of stenosing lesions of the great vessels in post mortem material. While the findings in any one case may be inconclusive from a large series, some definite trends should be established. Fisher, in 1951, stressed the importance of examining the neck vessels in cerebrovascular disease and the significance of this work led to further studies. Samuels, in 1956, reported his findings in 82 post mortem studies in which the neck arteries had been completely removed. There was a high incidence of atherosclerosis with stenoses and occlusions, with severe disease more common in males than females. Samuels was impressed by the consistent localization of these lesions and discussed the mechanical factors involved in their production. The most widely quoted of articles of this nature is the work of Hutchinson and Yates in 1957. The reason for its popularity by those espousing the great vessel basis for cerebrovascular disease is obvious from its content. The neck vessels were completely dissected in 83 patients dying of, or with a suggestive history of, cerebrovascular disease. In 40 of these patients, a significant stenosis or occlusion was present. The authors were convinced that the patients' clinical picture was due to progressive diminution in total cerebral blood flow and hemorrhage into an atheromatous plaque with elevation of the plaque and sudden increase in the degree of stenosis was considered a possible explanation for acute episodes in the course of the disease. Extracerebral factors were invoked in four cases in whom a cerebral infarct developed following a sudden drop in blood pressure. Since the areas of stenosis were quite localized, they believed that surgery on the neck vessels should be carried out with more frequency.

Another series with a more restrained conclusion was reported by Schwartz and Mitchel in 1961. They dissected the neck vessels from 93 unselected cases, most patients ranging in age from 55 to 75 and with only 27 dying of cerebrovascular disease. They found that 90% of men and 85% of women showed some degree of narrowing of the extracranial vessels and in 43% of men and 35% of women, this narrowing was severe. There were five cases with thrombotic occlusion, all of whom had cerebral infarcts. Although of the 27

patients with clinical stroke, 21 had narrowing of three or more
systems, in a significant proportion of patients over 75 with cerebrovascular symptoms, no stenosis was present in any part of the system.
They cautioned that, "without further evidence, one should not
necessarily conclude that the stroke is caused by the narrowing."

The post mortem study of Martin and colleagues was reviewed by
the same authors with clinical correlation. Although there was a
higher incidence of atherosclerosis of the neck arteries in those with
cerebrovascular disease than those dying of unrelated causes, they
concluded that although a relationship existed it was not necessarily
a direct one and that the demonstration of cervical stenosis or occlusions did not allow one to assume a positive relationship between
symptoms and the lesion. Radiographic studies of the extracranial
cerebral arteries were carried out on patients coming to post mortem
by Choi and Cromptom, and Stein and colleagues with a frequent
finding of unsuspected stenoses and occlusions. A clue to the intracranial components of cerebrovascular disease was given by the latter
authors in their conclusions, which is worth quoting: The — "most
significant factor was the incidence of severe intracranial atheromata
which was greater in the group with infarcts. This somewhat out-
weighed the significance of atheromatous involvement of the extracranial vessels which was also greater in the infarct group."

One pertinent study approached from the opposite direction was
carried out on healthy prison inmates by Faris and colleagues from
the University of Kansas. In 43 healthy men ranging in age from
40 to 65, arterial abnormalities were present on angiograms of the
neck vessels in 22%. A group of 68 male patients with cerebrovascular symptoms in the same age group showed similar abnormalities in 40%. In two of the 43 healthy men, there were complete
occlusions and in six, on turning the head, there was occlusion of one
of the vertebral arteries. They concluded that "the presence of certain
occlusive lesions in the vascular channels to the brain becomes of
critical importance only when other factors are radically altered."

The previous studies can be summarized very briefly by stating that,
although there is a higher incidence of occlusive disease of the neck
arteries in patients with cerebrovascular disease than in those without,
the difference is not great enough to warrant a cause and effect rela-

tionship in any one particular case. The equation remains indeterminate.

One easily-measured variable of importance in association with great vessel disease is the systemic blood pressure. That symptoms may be produced by hypotension in some cases with occlusive processes in the neck vessels has been repeatedly demonstrated, and symptoms appearing after hemorrhage, myocardial infarct, or vasodilator drugs are well known. We have seen a definite worsening of hemiparesis from a simple vagal reaction, due to apprehension prior to angiography. (This might be considered one of Baum's complications of "no" arteriography.) However, these reactions are not consistent. Hypotension for various causes occurs occasionally in patients undergoing neuroradiological investigation for cerebrovascular disease with no untoward reactions in the vast majority. Loeb, in a series of patients with a previous history of cerebrovascular episodes, found no neurological changes when the blood pressure was dropped to half its normal level.

Occlusive disease involving the great vessels arising from the aortic arch is apparently not as rare as previously thought. Rob quotes Broadbent as describing this entity in 1875 but it is better known as "Pulseless disease" or Takayusu's disease, from the Japanese Ophthalmologist who published an account in 1905, this being one of the earlier of many basic contributions made by ophthalmologists to the field of cerebral circulation. The surgical approach to these lesions was described by DeBakey and his colleagues in 1959. Although the occlusive process may involve any of the major trunks and was named from its effect in obliterating carotid and radial pulses, it is currently best known under the condition of one subclavian being occluded proximally, blood reaching the occluded segment by flowing down the vertebral artery on that side. This has been popularized as the "subclavian steal" and was described by Contorni in 1960 and by Reivich *et al.* in 1961. The effects of this "steal" are in diverting blood from the brain with symptomatology depending on how much is diverted from the vertebrobasilar system and how well the carotids are able to compensate. Chase and Kricheff found the subclavian steal in 5% of their arteriographic examinations of the aortic arch and in about half the cases the classical signs and symptoms were absent indicating not only that the condition is fairly common but also that the clinical diagnosis may be far from obvious. In our opinion, the greatest usefulness of the aortic arch study lies in the diagnosis of occlusive processes of this nature.

Any discussion of the role of large vessel disease would be incomplete without mentioning the role of kinking and coiling of the carotid arteries in the production of symptoms. The basic principles of hemodynamics indicate that at best these conditions would not be conducive to optimum blood flow and would predispose to turbulence and atheroma formation. Coiling is frequently found in children and is a developmental condition as opposed to kinking which is generally assumed to be degenerative. The problem was studied in some depth by Weibels and Fields in 1965. After reviewing their cases with coiling and kinking, they concluded that symptoms rarely occurred with coiling unless atherosclerotic occlusive disease was also present. With kinking, narrowing of the lumen was present in about half the cases and appeared to be related to atheroma formation rather than the degree of kinking itself. Symptoms of insufficiency appeared to be related to this narrowing in 10 of 33 cases leading to the conclusion that insufficiency was most likely precipitated because of failure of collateral circulation for one of several possible causes. Although the authors do not so state, it appears that the significance of kinking belongs in the same general category as stenosing lesions without kinking, the significance in any one case remaining an open question.

The history of the association of kinking and symptoms is interesting in that it is an excellent example of how the importance of diseases of the extracranial cerebral arteries has been exaggerated by inference and suggestion without factual misrepresentation, and in most cases in the absence of any direct statement by the authors themselves. The following excerpts from the literature illustrate the process.

In 1956, Hsu and Kistin stated that buckling of the great vessels was benign and surgery not indicated. Metz and colleagues at Queen Square, London, reviewed a thousand angiograms and found 161 with kinking of the carotids. From the association of cerebrovascular disease in the kinking as compared to the nonkinked, they concluded that with severe kinking there was a "strong suggestion" — not statistically significant — that the kinking predisposed to stroke. Derrick and Smith, quoting Metz' findings, say of the occurrence of cerebro-vascular disease with kinking, "the relations of this finding have become apparent." The article by Derrick and Smith was abstracted in *Modern Medicine*, the first sentence reading "kinking of the carotid artery is a common cause of cerebral insufficiency." The evolution, then, has gone from a negative (Hsu) to a "strong suggestion" (Metz) to "apparent" (Derrick) to an established dictum (Abstract).

SMALL EMBOLI IN THE PRODUCTION OF TRANSIENT ISCHEMIC ATTACKS

AN ALTERNATIVE CAUSE for symptoms described as cerebrovascular insufficiency or transient ischemic attacks is that of showers of small emboli usually arising from ulcerated plaques in the extracranial cerebral vessels. The embolic concept was suggested by Pickering in 1948 as an alternative to the theories of spasm. Although he suggested the heart as the source of emboli, this might have been given more attention but for the enthusiasm with which Denny-Brown's concept, relating insufficiency to extracranial stenoses and occlusions, was received. Before the embolic concept could be accepted, it was necessary to establish three facts: (1) that such emboli did occur and could be demonstrated; (2) that they might produce only transient symptoms, and (3) that they might repeatedly involve

———————→

5. SMALL EMBOLI AS A CAUSE OF TRANSIENT ISCHEMIC ATTACKS

   This 45-year-old man had a single stroke-like episode with no residua. An aortic arch study showed normal vessels except for a questionable abnormality in the one carotid and consequently, a direct carotid angiogram was done. The intracranial arteries were normal but there is an irregularity in the carotid sinus (see film) with the characteristic appearance of a mural thrombus.

   Emboli arising from a thrombus such as this are a common cause of transient ischemic attacks, especially in younger patients, and the intracranial vessels are usually normal. Emboli large or numerous enough to cause angiographic changes intracranially would also be expected to produce a more lasting neurological deficit.

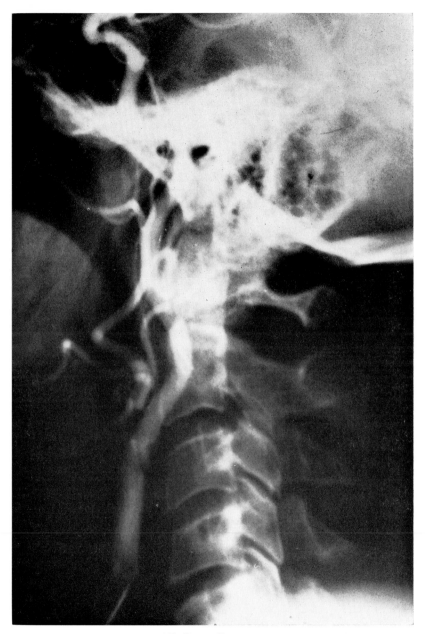

5. SMALL EMBOLI

While an open source of emboli to the brain is a hazardous and potentially fatal situation, the findings of Gunning and colleagues in England indicates that mural thrombi may heal spontaneously by becoming incorporated in the vessel wall. Unfortunately, at present there is no way of predicting what will happen in any individual case.

the same brain area. The facts were established in somewhat reverse order. Fisher and Adams, in 1951, found that emboli might cause an obstruction of an intracranial artery with subsequent lysis and fragmentation. Subsequent work in preventing transient ischemic attacks by anticoagulant therapy and angiographic observations of reopening of occluded vessels were confirmatory evidence. Since the emboli do not necessarily cause a permanent occlusion and the smaller ones may disappear very rapidly, their occurrence was not inconsistent with transient symptoms. Experimental work on monkeys by Denny-Brown and Meyer showed that experimentally-produced platelet emboli repeatedly lodged in the same vascular area and finally the identification of these small emboli was possible by seeing them in the fundus of the eye. Although this was reported as far back as 1875 by Gowers, its importance was revived by current reports such as those by Fisher an 1959, Hollenhorst in 1961, and the correlation of visible emboli with transient ischemic attacks described by Richardson and co-authors in 1962. A detailed account of the background and current status of the concept of small emboli was given by Millikan in 1965.

The composition as well as size of these emboli is important. The transient episodes appear due to the "white" emboli, made up mainly of platelets, that disintegrate much more rapidly than the predominantly fibrin emboli arising from a long standing thrombus, as in the left auricle. Embolization of atheromatous and calcific material from an ulcerated plaque, being resistant to lysis, would be expected to cause symptoms of longer duration although these, when seen in the retina, may also eventually disappear. This does not imply that all intravascular aggregates of platelets are embolic as they may be formed locally by stasis and Romanul and Abramowicz considered them the mechanism of small infarcts in the Denny-Brown type of insufficiency.

One objection to the embolic concept as opposed to the more popular thought of hemodynamic crisis associated with stenoses was encountered in personal experience, this being the fact that at endarterectomy on patients with a history of episodes suggesting transient ischemic attacks, the area of stenosis was often found smooth and devoid of thrombotic material. The explanation, not available at the time of the objection, was supplied by the two articles of Gunning and co-authors in 1964 in which they showed, first in the subclavian and later in the carotid arteries, that mural thrombi might give rise to emboli and subsequently become incorporated in the vessel wall. In their carotid series six patients without symptoms of retinal or cerebral ischemia for seven weeks or longer prior to surgery showed smooth laminated fibrin without recent thrombus at the site of stenoses.

CURRENT CONCEPTS OF INTRACRANIAL OCCLUSIONS

T HE CONCEPT OF small emboli as a cause of some cases of transient ischemic attacks has not been as generally accepted as would seem warranted in view of the facts. This is probably due to a reluctance to deviate from the popular belief that such episodes are due to hemodynamic crises associated with extracranial stenoses and occlusions. Denny-Brown, the originator of this concept, realized that the role of great vessel disease was being over-emphasized and wrote in 1960, "like many terms introduced into medicine, insufficiency has been used in a wider sense than that for which it was originally intended." The article continues that while hemodynamic crises associated with extracranial stenoses and occlusions are a common mechanism of symptoms production they are not the only cause. The role of platelet emboli is discussed.

Intracranial occlusions have not been overlooked by serious investigators in the field of neurology or neurosurgery, although all investigators have been hampered by the difficulties in demonstrating the intracranial processes. A surgeon might be expected to favor theories emphasizing the need for the surgical approach; however, Gurdjian, one of the early investigators in the surgical treatment of extracranial stenoses, wrote in 1961, "We should not be confused by the presence of atheromatous lesions in the larger vessels and ascribe to them causative significance when the real cause of disability is another type of vascular lesion or a concomittant nonvascular lesion." In other publications, Gurdjian and his group have repeatedly stated that in their belief the majority of strokes are due to intracranial occlusions. However, an earlier paper with Webster entitled "Observations on Hemiplegia with Middle Cerebral Artery Trunk Occlusion and with 'Normal' Carotid Angiogram," has been used as an argument that extracranial factors must be the more important since nothing is seen inside the head! The quotations around the word "normal" apparently were overlooked. What the article actually said was that the hemiplegia "may be due to involvement of smaller branches supplying the internal capsule or a more widespread involvement of the small branches of the middle cerebral artery supplying the cortex and subcortex."

The demonstration of the "border zone" infarcts has served to focus attention to intracranial components of this specific type, but since such infarcts are commonly secondary to severe extracranial stenosing lesions, the effect is to further emphasize the role of the extracranial vessels.

Radiologists, by adapting the catheter techniques to the aortic arch study, may have contributed to the overemphasis on the great vessels but in most cases, at least, not intentionally. Baker emphasized the necessity for complete intracranial studies in cerebrovascular disease. Cronqvist, in a correlative study between aortocervical and selective cerebral angiography, concluded that, "intracranial changes are more frequent than hitherto reported." Bull, with a long interest in the radiologic investigation of stroke, stressed the complexities and vast extent of the intracranial arteries and believed the normal angiogram in stroke patients was due to inability to recognize the lesion since angiography is, as he stated, a relatively crude procedure. Taveras, in clinical and postmortem material, has emphasized the intracranial factors. Newton, in describing four vessel arteriography in a popular journal at a time this study was at its zenith of popularity, might have been expected to emphasize the importance of the vessels under consideration. Instead, he conservatively stated that extracranial occlusive processes were a "common cause" of cerebrovascular insufficiency.

Pathologists are usually considered to be the final judge of disease processes and recent studies should leave no doubt as to the frequency of intracranial occlusions. Winter and Gyori, in 1960, found the site

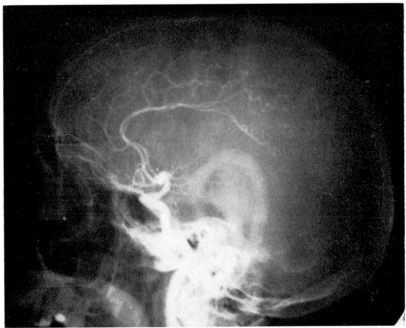

6. COMPLETE OCCLUSION OF THE MIDDLE CEREBRAL ARTERY

Gross occlusions of the major intracranial arteries are not a problem in angiographic diagnosis. However, occlusion of the individual branches are five times as common as the occlusion of the main trunk of the middle cerebral artery shown in this illustration.

of occlusion in 19 of 21 brains that had evidence of small infarcts. The discrepancy between this and earlier reports in which no intracranial occlusion were found in large numbers of cases is explained by the authors as follows: ". . . the examination of the vessels is difficult and time consuming and therefore thorough examinations are rarely made." In a study of 178 routine postmortem examinations, Fisher and co-authors found occlusions of the neck vessels in sixteen cases. However, intracranial occlusions were more frequently encountered, there being fourteen cases with intracranial arterial thrombosis, seventeen with embolic occlusions, nineteen with lacunae of previous infarcts and ten with infarcts of uncertain etiology. In addition, nineteen cases showed evidence of intracerebral hemorrhage. Moossy found intracranial arterial thromboses in 55% of 142 cerebral infarcts and stated that, "while this study does not diminish the importance of the extracranial carotid and vertebral arteries, it does tend to restore the intracranial arterial system to a position worthy of more consideration that it has enjoyed recently."

The rare form of progressive occlusions of children and young adults that involves the proximal intracerebral arteries and seems more common in the Japanese can best be classified as an arteritis.

MECHANICS OF OCCLUSIVE CEREBROVASCULAR DISEASE

THE CLASSIFICATION of symptoms produced by occlusive cerebro-vascular disease with terms such as "transient ischemic attack," "incipient stroke," and "completed stroke" are excellent tools for the clinician but likely to be confusing to the radiologist. Systems of classification such as the recent one by Heyman, in general, tended to follow clinical rather than anatomical lines. The following outline of causes for the disease processes is anatomical and mechanistic and conceived through the viewpoint of a radiologist. It is included here merely to summarize the processes that should be considered in the angiographic investigation of the stroke patient.

1. Extracranial Stenoses and Occlusions
   A. Abrupt occlusions of any extracranial cerebral artery causing brain infarction by itself.
      This is a time-honored concept, especially when carotid occlusion is concerned, but the frequency with which neurosurgical patients have tolerated ligation of the carotid for therapeutic purposes suggests that this should not be frequent and would be expected to occur only when the anatomy of the circle of Willis precludes immediate collateral or when there is an associated intracranial occlusion concealed by the proximal one. We have been especially interested in this phenomenon.
   B. A gradual stenoses or occlusion of one or more extracranial arteries giving rise to episodic cerebral dysfunction.

[30]

Under these conditions, collateral circulation develops so efficiently that ordinarily the brain is adequately perfused and the patient is essentially normal. Under some circumstances, often associated with systemic factors such as anemia, hemorrhage, reduced cardiac output, vasodilator drugs or a drop in blood pressure from any cause, the collateral is insufficient and the patient develops temporary cerebral ischemia with symptoms resulting. If the ischemia is sufficiently severe or prolonged, infarcts may develop. Diminution of flow by "pinching" the extracerebral vessels on turning the head is thought to have the same effect. This is the hemodynamic crisis and insufficiency of Denny-Brown and is a very real and well documented entity. Our only quarrel with this concept is that it has been so exaggerated in many quarters that it is accepted as the only important cause of stroke.

C. Atheromatous areas in the extracranial cerebral arteries giving rise to emboli.

   1) From ulcerations on the vessel wall showers of platelet emboli may arise giving rise to cerebral and/or occular symptoms. Since these emboli are rapidly lysed, the symptoms are transitory.

   2) Larger emboli of thrombotic material cause intracranial occlusions that, due to larger vessels involved and a relatively slow lysis, cause brain infarcts and permanent changes.

   3) Atheromatous and calcific debris may embolize from the sudden evacuation of an atheromatous plaque, symptoms depending on size and extent of embolization. The only problem associated with this mechanism is that the atheromata responsible for the emboli are often seen as narrowings in the arterial lumen and the symptoms attributed to the narrowing, even if slight, as under B above.

D. Occlusions of the thoracic trunks, as in A and B, or reversal of vertebral blood flow, depleting cerebral circulation in the "subclavian steal."

E. Combinations of the above—occlusions, stenoses and emboli.

F. Extracranial stenoses and occlusions may be incidental findings not associated with neurological symptoms or brain infarctions.

2. Intracranial Lesions
   A. Atherosclerotic occlusions.
   B. Generalized intracerebral arteriosclerosis without occlusions of visible vessels.
   C. Primary thromboses, usually associated with atherosclerosis.
   D. Intracranial emboli from any source.
   E. Intracranial occlusions not necessarily associated with arteriosclerosis including the arteritides, migraine, blood abnormalities or parasitic infestations such as the cerebral manifestations of malaria.

   The concept of stress, leading to increased coagulability of the blood as a factor in stroke as suggested by Davis, belongs in this category as would the effects of the "pill" if one accepts this as an established fact.
   F. Occlusions secondary to other intracranial processes such as pressure from tumors, oedema, hematomata or infectious processes.

   The fact that infarcts, by the resultant edema, can result in occlusion of other vessels has been noted by us angiographically and demonstrated in brain specimens by Sohn and Levine.
   G. Functional occlusions in the presence of patent vessels due to shunting as in AV malformations, fistulae or highly vascular tumors.
   H. Combinations of the above, especially an underlying atherosclerosis with conditions favoring thrombosis.
3. Combination of Extracranial and Intracranial Occlusions, "Concealed" Occlusions

   As previously mentioned, intracranial occlusions, either embolic or thrombotic, may occur in conjunction with extracranial ones and unless there is good filling of intracranial vessels by external carotid collateral or the non-occluded extracranial vessels are studied, the intracranial occlusions are never seen.
4. External Carotid Occlusions

   A theoretical consideration might be involvement of the external carotids, either by arteriosclerotic occlusions, surgical ligation or tumorous involvement, or functional occlusions by involvement in AV malformations or even severe Paget's disease, depriving the patient of collateral developed in the presence of occlusive processes of the internal carotid or vertebral arteries and so being directly responsible for the development of stroke. It seems likely that this does occur but to our knowledge has not been reported as such. (The report by Hardesty documenting just such a condition appeared as this work was going to press.)

INCIDENCE AND SIGNIFICANCE OF SMALL VESSEL OCCLUSION

THE POSSIBLE MECHANISMS for the production of occlusive cerebro-vascular disease as outlined can probably be accepted by most physicians as valid since no one believes that intracranial occlusions do not occur. The point of difference lies in a belief as to their incidence and significance. These two are closely related in practice since those who assume them to be of no practical significance are hardly interested in the frequency with which they occur. Unfortunately, this view point seems to predominate at this time and, as compared to the vast sums spent on investigation of other aspects of cerebrovascular disease, there has been little encouragement for detailed investigation of the intracranial components. In a round table discussion of the cerebral circulation in Paris, Gautier, in commenting on this problem, described the investigation of intracranial occlusions as the "poor relative" of research.

The percentage of strokes caused by small intracranial occlusions can only be estimated. In our experience, they were found in 15% of all cases with angiographically proven occlusive cerebrovascular disease. When selecting cases on the basis of a discharge diagnosis of cerebral thrombosis or embolism, the percentage is somewhat lower, one reason being that we do not consider generalized intracranial arteriosclerosis as angiographic proof of occlusive processes. Since cerebral angiography is not routine at this institution, these figures are biased and favor more patients with possible surgical lesions of the extracranial arteries. As compared to other common cerebrovascular occlusions, we have found branch occlusions about half as often as internal carotid thrombosis and five times as often as complete occlusion of the middle cerebral artery. When both complete and partial middle cerebral artery occlusions are considered, the partial corresponding to what we classify as multiple branch occlusions, these were found to occur in about the same number as occlusions of isolated branches. Considering occlusions of the smaller branches as a whole, about three-quarters involve the middle cerebral artery with the pericallosals being next in frequency. We have seen relatively few occlusions of branches of the posterior cerebral arteries but since these fill in less than a third of carotid angiograms and studies of the basilar circulation are not done as often as those of the carotids, this is not a true picture. In this area, we have diagnosed occlusions as often by seeing retrograde filling as by finding absence of branches.

Despite the lack of accurate statistics, it can be said that small intracranial occlusions are common events. Since they are common, they cannot be dismissed as unimportant because there is no direct treatment comparable to carotid endarterectomy. If for no other reason, they should be recognized for the sake of medical accuracy merely because they exist. Development of effective means of prevention and treatment of cerebrovascular disease must be on a factual basis and include all aspects of the process irrespective of their current popularity.

There are practical as well as philosophical reasons for recognizing these small occlusions and one of them lies in the realm of treatment already available.

In 1963, Fazekas, Alman and Sullivan described the difficulties in determining which patients would benefit from endarterectomy for occlusive processes in the extracranial arteries. In the same journal issue, the problem was discussed by Millikan in an editorial with the same conclusions which were, in effect, that it was impossible to select in advance those who would be improved by surgery as opposed to those who would not. By contrast, at the 1967 Symposium Neuroradiologicum, Wood, in describing experience with patients following reconstructive surgery on the neck vessels stated that those with transient ischemic attacks due to embolization from the involved arterial segment had no further attacks and had remained completely well during the period of observation.

It is equally helpful to be able to make a definitive diagnosis. We accept a diagnosis of generalized intracranial arteriosclerosis with reluctance since it is not definitive. If one can point out an occlusion to explain the patient's symptomatology, the possibility of early malignant gliomas or metastatic brain lesions is highly unlikely and the patient may be spared the time and expense of repeated studies.

There are other "fringe benefits" from an accurate diagnosis—the arterial changes indicative of an arteritis which is a systemic rather than a local cerebral disease is one. Prognosis is another. In our experience, patients with isolated branch occlusions do well and would benefit from early ambulation, rehabilitation and reassurance. Pasteur did some of his most brilliant work after suffering a "small" stroke.

The relationship between cardiac disease manifested primarily by pulmonary edema with intracranial processes is a fascinating one that will undoubtedly receive more attention. ECG changes following brain injury have been reported from this institution by Falsetti and Moody and, more recently, Blum and colleagues found that irreversible myocardial infarcts developed in otherwise healthy monkeys after repeated stimulation of the insula. The possible role of occlusive cerebrovascular disease in producing such changes has not been established as yet but this should be possible in the future.

SECTION 9

DIAGNOSIS OF SMALL VESSEL OCCLUSION

IF ONE AGREES that intracranial occlusions are important, it becomes necessary to make the diagnosis. This can be done in the majority of cases by making full use of the information available on cerebral angiograms. The criteria used to diagnose occlusion of branches of the intracranial arteries can be summarized as follows:

Direct Evidence
1. A visible point of obstruction in the occluded vessel.
2. Absence of a vessel in its usual location, not explainable by anatomical or technical factors.

Indirect Evidence
A. Diagnostic: Retrograde filling of an occluded branch
B. Nondiagnostic but suggestive or confirmatory
   1. Local stasis of contrast material
   2. A capillary blush or prominent small vessels in the area of occlusion
   3. Early drainage veins from the same area
   4. Edema in the area of occlusion

The direct evidence of arterial occlusion is the same as that applied in the leg, arm or abdomen, the only differences are in the anatomy of the areas involved. The three dimensional course of the intra-cranial arteries, particularly the branches of the middle cerebral artery, as they dip in and out of the sulci or are enfolded in the insula while

[37]

at the same time continuing their linear course, results in considerable overlap that frequently conceals the actual point of obstruction. This is unavoidable although careful correlation of all projections may be helpful as occasionally the stump of an occluded artery may be seen in the frontal rather than the lateral projection. The use of stereoscopic angiography, by producing two slightly different projections, may increase the likelihood of silhouetting the point of obstruction but, at best, in many cases this is never seen. There are reasons for this, both anatomical and physiological. Occlusions, either from thrombosis or lodgement of emboli, tend to occur at the site of branching of vessels. An occlusion distal to such branching often results in a retrograde thrombosis due to stasis of blood back to the point where free blood flow is possible. The one remaining patent branch then appears to be a normal continuation of the vessel, its sudden change of course quite normal for a cortical artery and the occluded branch simply disappears.

Absence of a vessel in its usual location is generally accepted as angiographic proof of occlusion in all parts of the body except the head. Some years ago, eminent neuroradiologists stated that this was not a reliable criterion in cerebral angiography and this opinion was recently reaffirmed by Lee and Hodes. In speaking of the middle cerebral artery, they stated: "The absence of one of its major vessels may be a congenital anomaly and not due to occlusion." Although disagreeing completely with this statement, there is some factual basis for it that is worth discussing. If attention is limited to the arteries in the Sylvian fissure, it is undoubtedly true that "absence" of a vessel may be due to a variant rather than to disease. Except in the simplest anatomical arrangements, trying to identify the arteries proximally and tracing them to their termination is difficult or impossible. To appreciate the normalcy of the numerous variations in the Sylvian vessels, it is helpful even if not correct and at best a gross oversimplication, to consider the developing brain as if the arteries were completely pre-formed and following the brain through its differential growth with rotation, bending and enfolding. The arteries must elongate between their two fixed points—origin and termination. If elongation takes place at the origin, one may expect one main trunk giving off the various branches. If elongation is distal, the parent vessel divides into a number of separate arteries near its source, in this case at the mouth of the Sylvian fissure. With this picture in mind, the numerous variations in the Sylvian vessels are to be expected and need not cause undue confusion.

If one considers the areas of termination of these branches, congenital absence of any one, if it occurs at all, must be exceedingly rare. In dissection of vessels of over 150 brains and tracings of over 500 normal carotid angiograms by Doctor Waddington and myself, we have never encountered congenital absence of any branches of the middle cerebral artery. In clinical material, we have seen absence of branches in children which may have been either congenital or perhaps more likely acquired in utero or the neonatal period. However, in either case they resulted in a very definite cerebral abnormality of both structure and function.

The important fact is that every portion of the brain has a constant blood supply irrespective of the course or point of origin of the supplying artery. This is the key to the diagnosis of small vessel occlusion and cannot be over-emphasized. If those interested in angiographic diagnosis in cerebrovascular disease get nothing more from this book than the habit of looking at the termination rather than the origin of the intracerebral arteries, their diagnostic acumen will be improved.

The only indirect evidence of occlusion of an intracranial branch that is diagnostic is retrograde filling of the occluded branch. The retrograde filling is made possible by the pial anastomotic network and when larger vessels are involved may be very prominent. The difficulties in depending on this finding for a diagnosis may be summarized as follows:

1) It is not always present.
2) Retrograde filling may be present but not obvious when small arteries are involved.
3) Delayed filling, due to technical factors or an incomplete occlusion, may be confused with retrograde filling.

Reliable figures as to the frequency of retrograde filling in the presence of occlusion are not available and will vary with the criteria used to make the diagnosis of occlusion and also the effort expended in finding it. This retrograde filling has a physiological as well as an anatomical basis and does not necessarily occur and persist merely because an occlusion is present. Laroche and Cronqvist found that early drainage veins or a capillary blush did not occur when collateral circulation was seen. The frequency of visible collateral may vary with the timing of the angiographic examination. In our experience, this seems to develop early and is frequently obvious in the presence of occlusions of major trunks or of one artery that supplies more than one branch such as the ascending frontal complex but not when the occlusion involves a small and distal vessel. The radiographic density of vessels filled by intracranial collateral is often less than that in arteries filled directly and this reduced density, plus a vessel size of a millimeter or less, makes recognition difficult. Retrograde filling may occur and has been demonstrated even in very small branches but as a rule this can be done only by careful search after the diagnosis of occlusion has been made. Although occasionally helpful as confirmatory evidence, retrograde filling of small vessels occluded distally is of little practical value as a primary diagnostic sign.

Delayed filling due to technical factors or stenoses of intracranial vessels may be confused with retrograde filling but should not be if serial films are available and observed in sequence, this being merely a matter of determining whether the contrast is coming or going.

In our experience, the greatest value of retrograde filling of occluded arteries is in diagnosing an occlusion of an artery that is not filled directly. This has been very effective in the diagnosis of posterior cerebral and basilar artery occlusions when the posterior cerebral did not fill from the carotids. The same applies to occlusions of the anterior cerebral or proximal pericallosal arteries since nonfilling from one side is often normal and is not diagnostic unless both sides are studied.

Of the three nondiagnostic but confirmatory findings, stasis is the most valuable although it is quite nonspecific. Stasis may result from pressure on normal vessels and has not been a common finding in our series of isolated branch occlusions, probably because the portion of the vessel just proximal to the occlusion that would be expected to show the stasis soon becomes completely thrombosed. We have noted stasis most often and found it of greatest value in cases with multiple emboli. This is probably due to two factors—first, emboli tend to be recurrent and we probably see very recent occlusions with stasis before either the proximal portion of the vessel has had time to thrombose or the embolus has lysed sufficiently to move on. Secondly, either multiple micro-emboli or fragmentation and partial lysis of a larger embolus may occlude many of the tiny distal ramifications of a branch, leaving the visible portion of the artery intact but partially plugging its run-off. The findings of stasis in one area, not explainable by local edema or a mass lesion, plus a definite occlusion or local stasis in several areas not explainable by other mechanisms, is characteristic of emboli.

The capillary blush and early drainage veins might be expected in occlusive processes on the basis of the hyperemia around the ischemic area shown by Meyer and Denny-Brown in 1957 and more recently by Waltz and Sundt. Although only recently publicized, these changes have been recognized for some time and were described by Woringer and colleagues in 1958. The greatest problem with the capillary blush is one of definition, this being a rather vague term and from the discussion at the VIIIth Symposium Neuroradiologicum it appears there is some disagreement as to what does and what does not constitute a capillary blush. Certainly, a blushlike appearance is a common pressure effect and not necessarily related to occlusions and its prominence will vary with circulation time and the amount of contrast employed. Frequently, vessels at the site of occlusion that are ordinarily too small to be seen become dilated from collateral flow and give a characteristic appearance even though in our opinion it is hardly "blush" like. Early drainage veins are quite definite but have been found in a variety of conditions and are most often manifestations of malignant gliomas. Steven, in a paper given in 1959, before the relationship of early venous filling and occlusions were appreciated, described this finding as one of the pitfalls of the angiographic diagnosis of tumor. At best, a capillary blush and early drainage veins are findings that can be used as confirmatory evidence of occlusion only when the diagnosis of occlusion is established by other means.

Edema about infarcts cause by small occlusions is not of much diagnostic help since it is quite variable. At times, by pushing the surrounding vessels away from the infarct, it makes the avascular area more prominent, but at other times it is only confusing. In general, vascular displacement associated with the smaller occlusions is not at all pronounced, but there are exceptions in which the degree of edema seems out of proportion to the size of the vessel involved and the resultant displacement may suggest a tumor or intracerebral hematoma. One can say that minimal vascular displacement is not inconsistent with an occlusion.

Other diagnostic procedures and findings can only be mentioned in passing. Pneumoencephalography may be diagnostic in localizing an intracerebral hematoma or discovering a central tumor masquerading as vascular disease. In our experience, the spinal fluid examination has usually been normal. Electroencephalograms are usually abnormal but only occasionally are the changes well localized. We have been impressed with the value of serial isotopic brain scanning as, when positive, this localizes the area very well and the radioactive uptake diminishes with time as opposed to the findings in tumors that become progressively more definite. Since gliomas may simulate cerebrovascular disease before they are large enough to be obvious on angiograms, this is of practical significance. A single negative brain scan does not exclude an occlusion, as the isotope is only concentrated in the area at a certain point in the evolution of the infarct. Good clinical correlation that is very satisfying to the clinician is possible in most cases of isolated branch occlusion. Although the precise syndromes described by Foix and Levy have fallen into disrepute, this is the fault of angiographic diagnosis rather than lack of specificity of brain areas. The difficulties commonly encountered are in cases with gross occlusions or those involving multiple areas where the findings are, as stated by Lascelles and Burrows, "lost in the massive neurological deficit that customarily occurs." This is especially likely to occur with embolic processes as they are usually multiple and changes arising from small occlusions in motor areas may completely mask occlusions of larger vessels elsewhere. If, however, an isolated branch is involved confirmatory clinical findings are to be expected.

ANATOMY OF THE INTRACRANIAL ARTERIES

Since the areas supplied by the intracranial arteries, especially the middle cerebral, is constant and the absence of a vessel the most consistent finding in the presence of occlusion, the diagnosis rests primarily on the ability to recognize the absence of branches in any particular area. In some cases, by simply looking at the normal areas of vascular distribution, the diagnosis is obvious without any other knowledge of anatomy. Unfortunately, it is not always that simple—if it were, the diagnosis could be made by a draftsman and a computer. The zones that can be applied to the area of the middle cerebral artery by artificial lines are an aid and not a substitute for anatomic study.

The anatomy of the supratentorial arteries is divided into sections in order of their importance, the middle, pericallosal and posterior cerebral. The choroidal and penetrating arteries have been studied in detail by others and are not included.

Middle Cerebral Artery

If one refers to textbooks of neuroanatomy, the branches of the middle cerebral artery are given a variety of names that differ from one author to another and even between text and illustrations in the same book. For angiographic purposes, the branches are generally described as four main trunks, the ascending frontal or ascending frontoparietal, posterior parietal, angular and posterior temporal. The ascending frontal is as large as the rest combined and is customarily

[43]

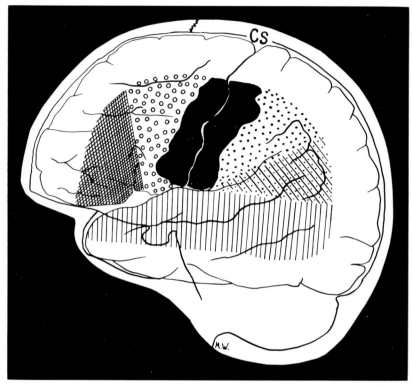

7. SCHEMATIC DRAWING OF LATERAL ASPECT OF THE CEREBRAL
HEMISPHERE

Although the template applied to the branches of the middle cerebral
artery was developed empirically, the reason it is effective is that it is anatomical
as shown in the drawing. The zones are outlined by various shadings, these
being, from left to right, the orbitofrontal, operculofrontal and central sulcus
areas of the ascending frontal complex, followed by the posterior parietal,
angular and temporal areas. The shading employed is used to identify individual branches in subsequent illustrations and the central sulcus arteries in
solid black are usually included as landmarks in drawings of the pericallosal
vessels.

treated as a unit. However, Lima divides this complex into three
divisions, essentially the same as employed here, which are the orbitofrontal, operculofrontal or candelabra, and the arteries in the central
sulcus.

The anatomic descriptions following are based on dissections of
over 150 adult brains and tracings of over 500 normal carotid angiograms and is a composite of studies previously published.

The middle cerebral artery arises from one main trunk at the "T" junction of the internal carotid. Very rarely (less than 0.1%), it may arise as two or more separate vessels. The small penetrating arteries are given off posteriorly and in about the same location the anterior temporal artery arises, sending tiny twigs down over the temporal pole and a recurrent branch that runs posteriorly supplying the anterior lateral aspect of the temporal lobe. The main trunk of the middle cerebral artery in the majority of cases gives off one or more major branches proximal to the mouth of the Sylvian fissure, these most commonly being the posterior temporal and/or part of the

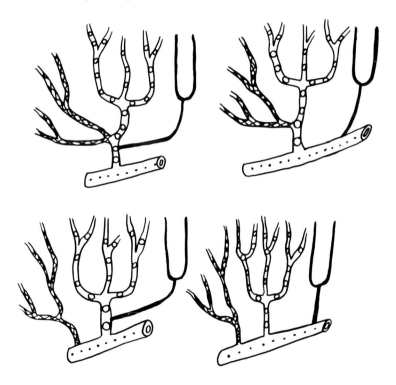

8. PATTERNS OF ASCENDING FRONTAL COMPLEX

The ascending frontal complex, with its three components shown in different shading, sometimes arises as a single trunk (*upper left*), but more often as two trunks, with either the orbitofrontal or central sulcus arteries sharing one trunk with the operculofrontal (*upper right, lower left*). Occasionally, the three components have separate origins (*lower right*) and, in addition, not illustrated, various branches of the components may arise separately so that the ascending frontal complex takes off as four or five small arteries.

ascending frontal complex. The main artery breaks up into its branches at the mouth of the Sylvian fissure but seldom in a clear cut bi- or trifurcation. The number of main trunks in the Sylvian fissure distal to this point varies greatly. In the simplest case, there is only one that gives rise to the other branches while in the most complex there are separate trunks to every individual area, often with one or more smaller accessory branches in addition. In the majority, two main trunks are present.

The first major branch is the ascending frontal complex that we have divided into three components. These components can only be recognized by their distal course, as the origins of the first two are usually impossible to find angiographically and from dissections there is found to be a confusing variation. Occasionally, there is one short massive trunk giving rise to the three divisions and, at the other extreme, not only do the three divisions arise separately but branches of the divisions arise independently so that there is a series of small branches arising from a parent trunk. The most common arrangement is that of two components sharing one trunk of origin with the third arising independently.

Orbitofrontal Artery

The orbitofrontal branches supply the lateral portion of the orbital surface and the inferior and middle frontal gyri of the frontal lobe. They can be distinguished from the operculofrontal branches behind them in that they have a distinct anterior inclination (Fig. 16). In about half the cases, there are two or three branches of fair size— in the remainder, multiple smaller ones. These vessels are seen overlying and in front of the pericallosal arteries and are always big enough to be seen although their extent is quite variable since they vary inversely in size with the branches to adjoining areas from the pericallosal. When the frontopolar branch is small or absent, or often when both pericallosal arteries are filled from the opposite carotid, the orbitofrontal branches are large and extend up to the superior frontal gyrus. This occurs in about a third of the cases. Occlusion of this division as an isolated event is uncommon, it being the least frequently involved of all the major middle cerebral artery branches.

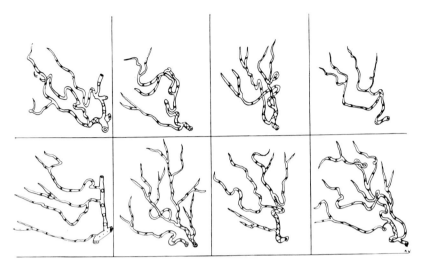

9. PATTERNS OF ORBITOFRONTAL ARTERIES

These eight drawings are tracings of the orbitofrontal branches taken from normal carotid angiograms. Since the pericallosal arteries tend to conceal these vessels, these cases were those in which the pericallosal artery was not filled and, as a result of this selection, the branches may be larger than average. The general course and distribution, however, is representative. While the course and origin of these branches is highly variable, the general area of distribution is constant. The definite anterior inclination of the vessels is characteristic and serves to separate them from the operculofrontal branches.

Operculofrontal or Candelabra Arteries

The operculofrontal or candelabra group are the arteries that are enfolded in the insula and after looping down from under the operculum to reach the lateral surface of the frontal lobe pass almost directly upward. This is the largest component of the ascending frontal complex and is responsible for the term "candelabra" that is often applied to the ascending frontal group as a whole. In nearly half the cases, this division is made up of three vessels that bifurcate fairly symmetrically to produce six terminal branches above the insula. With this anatomical arrangement, the term candelabra is quite descriptive. The next most common arrangement is that of two arteries that bifurcate and rebifurcate, and in the remainder there is a haphazard system of branching and rebranching so that there may be as many as ten terminal branches above the operculum.

Other vessels running up the Sylvian fissure occasionally have a high looping course in the same area and may tend to obscure absence of operculofrontal branches unless one looks for the distal ramifications.

Central Sulcus Artery

Either one or two arteries in the central sulcus (Rolandic fissure) is a constant finding although the origin of the vessels vary and, while we have included these vessels as part of the ascending frontal complex, this is not strictly true in all cases. In half the cases there are two arteries in the sulcus. If one is present, it is larger and

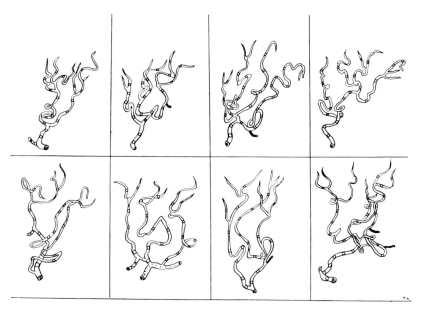

10. PATTERNS OF OPERCULOFRONTAL ARTERY

These are characteristic patterns of the operculofrontal artery traced from normal carotid angiograms. The most common arrangements are either three vessels that bifurcate or two vessels that bifurcate and rebifurcate. However, there are many variations of these basic patterns so this complex is best identified by its course. Proximally, these branches are folded under the operculum and so make characteristic loops as they come out from under the operculum. Distally, their course is primarily upward as opposed to the anterior inclination of the orbitofrontal branches and the posterior inclination of the arteries in the central sulcus.

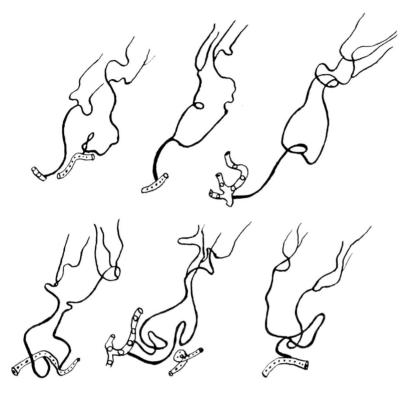

11. PATTERN OF CENTRAL SULCUS ARTERIES

These drawings are tracings from angiograms representing the common forms of the central sulcus artery(ies). There are two about as often as one, both arising from the same or different trunks in approximately equal numbers. It is important to remember that if a single artery is present, it invariably bifurcates so that a single central sulcus artery, without major branching, is only seen as a result of an occlusion. Although the arteries, or the two branches if one is present, undulate considerably in the depths of the fissure, it is usually not difficult to estimate the axis of the central sulcus from the course of the vessels. The characteristic loop of the artery as it goes around the posterior lip of the operculum is seen in several figures. An uncommon variant in which the artery enters the fissure above the level of the operculum is not shown.

invariably bifurcates and, whether there are two arteries or one with two branches, the anterior component supplies the motor and the posterior the sensory areas. When two arteries are present they may arise from the same or distinctly different parent trunks. One artery may have a separate origin proximally in the Sylvian fissure, arise

The Neglected Cause of Stroke

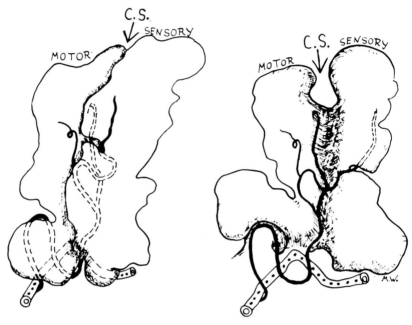

12. CHARACTERISTIC APPEARANCE OF CENTRAL SULCUS ARTERY AT
ITS ORIGIN

The central sulcus artery, when arising as the most posterior branch of the
operculofrontal vessels, has a characteristic appearance that will identify it
in over 50% of angiograms. The anatomical arrangement responsible for this
appearance is shown in the drawings. On the left, with the brain undisturbed,
the artery is seen under the operculum. It loops downward as the other operculofrontal branches, but also loops posteriorly to go around the posterior lip
of the operculum before entering the depths of the Rolandic fissure. The
drawing on the right shows the operculum elevated and the central sulcus
spread apart with the artery deep in the fissure sending the branches up to the
surface.

as part of the operculofrontal branch or independently from the most
superior trunk in the Sylvian fissure in the region of the central
sulcus. This trunk is ordinarily either the posterior parietal artery
or an artery that divides to become both posterior parietal and angular
arteries. When the central sulcus artery arises from the operculofrontal
branches, it takes a characteristic dip around the lip of the operculum
posteriorly as it goes into the depths of the fissure. The course of the
artery or arteries in the central sulcus is not necessarily a straight line
as the vessels may undulate considerably in the depths of the sulcus

and the branches coming to the surface may extend to the limits of both pre- and post-central gyri, covering an area fully an inch wide. The vessels in the central sulcus run deeper than other vessels and can be seen on angiograms in the frontal projection, provided there is sufficient angulation and good radiographic technique, as the most inferior of the middle cerebral branches that are directed medially (Fig. 18).

In about half the cases, the motor strip has an accessory blood supply from the operculofrontal branches that runs posteriorly on the cortical surface and can be seen approaching or crossing the central sulcus arteries that are in the depths of the fissure.

These vessels are of considerable importance since they outline the central sulcus and hence serve to identify the motor strip and their occlusion produces a pronounced neurological deficit with minimal angiographic change.

Posterior Parietal Artery

The posterior parietal artery commonly arises from a trunk that

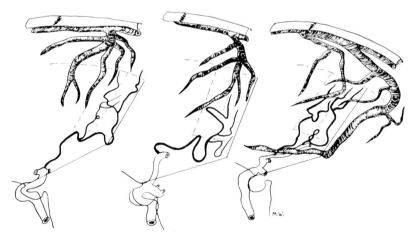

13. COURSE OF THE VEIN OF TROLARD IN RELATION TO THE CENTRAL SULCUS

The anastomatic vein of Trolard has long been used as an indicator of the position of the motor strip. The inaccuracy of this landmark is shown in the drawings. The vein was anterior to the central sulcus in about a fourth of 100 cases, posterior in another fourth, and corresponded to the central sulcus arteries in the remaining half.

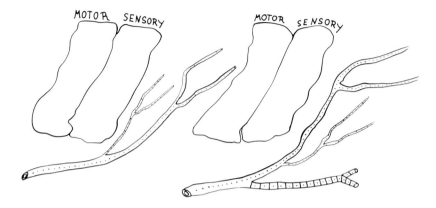

14. ACCESSORY PARIETAL ARTERY

An accessory artery to the posterior parietal area is found in 10% or more of individuals and may lead to confusion. This extra branch may be either anterior or posterior to the major artery and bears no relationship to the central sulcus arteries, being found in equal frequency with either one or two vessels in the central sulcus.

terminates as the angular. In general, it has a greater upward inclination than the angular and a greater posterior inclination than the axis of the central sulcus arteries. It would be angiographically very simple to recognize except for two facts: (1) its area is superimposed on the distal ramifications of the pericallosal artery, and (2) not infrequently there is an additional artery that may have a separate origin to the same area. The larger of the two may be either anterior or posterior to the extra branch and, while the terms "anterior" and "posterior parietal" arteries have been used, we believe it much simpler to stick with one name—posterior parietal—and call the intruder an accessory branch.

Angular Artery

The angular artery commonly shares its origin with the posterior parietal and is usually the larger of the two. In the most simple anatomical arrangements, it is often seen as the termination of the largest trunk running directly up the axis of the Sylvian fissure and has been called the "Terminal Artery." At the end of the fissure, the axis of the angular artery changes and is directly posterior in the long axis of the skull or with even a slight inferior inclination. When this vessel is large, its branches may overlap the areas of the posterior parietal above and the posterior temporal below.

Posterior Temporal Artery

The lateral surface of the temporal lobe presents a sizable area and perhaps it is unfortunate that by custom only one of the vessels supplying it is given angiographic recognition. On the other hand, this artery, the posterior temporal, is the only one that is at all consistent and of significant size. In about 60% of cases, this is a good sized branch that leaves the Sylvian fissure by means of a characteristic "hairpin" turn as it comes up from the fissure and goes down over the lateral surface. In about 15% of cases, the vessel is very large and leaves the Sylvian fissure near its mouth so that it simulates to some extent the course of the posterior cerebral.

It is impossible for one vessel to supply the entire area of the temporal lobe even when large. The anterior temporal branch supplies the temporal pole and a varying portion of the anterior lateral aspect. There are also anterior temporal branches from the posterior cerebral and the posterior cerebral itself supplies the inferior portion of the temporal lobe. There are accessory branches arising from various sources coming down over the lateral aspect of the temporal lobe between the areas supplied by the anterior temporal in front and the posterior temporal posteriorly. When the posterior temporal is small, and leaves the fissure distally, some of these may be of fair size and have been called "middle" temporal arteries. Since such prominent branches are present in only some 25% or less, we doubt that they warrant a name although their presence and significance should be appreciated. In about 5% of cases, there are multiple vessels to the temporal lobe area with none predominating enough to be given a specific name.

Although these variations would appear to make a diagnosis of posterior temporal artery occlusion very difficult, this does not seem to be the case. If one considers the area rather than the individual branches, it is surprisingly easy to mentally equate several small branches with one large one and to recognize a few tiny vessels and no large one as the result of an occlusion. The inverse size relationship of one branch to another in an adjoining area is especially prominent

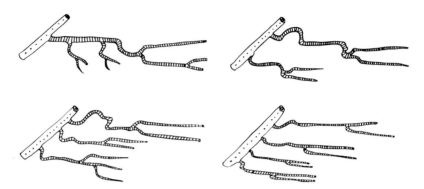

15. PATTERNS OF THE TEMPORAL BRANCHES OF THE MIDDLE CEREBRAL ARTERY

Common variations of the blood supply to the lateral temporal lobe are shown in these schematic figures. A single large posterior temporal artery (*upper left*) supplying the area by itself is found in some 15% while a smaller and more distal posterior temporal artery, associated with a good sized branch that might be called a "middle temporal" artery is found in about 25% (*upper right*). More often, there is more than one additional branch to the area (*lower left*) and rarely, there are multiple smaller vessels without any one predominating (*lower right*).

in the temporal area. A greater difficulty in diagnosing posterior temporal occlusions is caused by filling of the posterior cerebral as this tends to obscure the area.

Template

Artificial means of simplifying the intracranial vascular anatomy are not new. Fischer published a work in 1938 in which portions of the arteries were numbered and this was used by Ecker in his book, *The Normal Cerebral Angiogram*. The zonal concept of blood supply has also been used in a general way by others, including Greitz, and LaRoche and Cronqvist. These authors, however, were referring to venous drainage rather than the arteries themselves. LaRoche and Cronqvist utilized the areas where early drainage veins occurred, plus other findings, as a method of determining arterial occlusions. The zonal approach used here is the same in principle although since it deals with the arteries themselves, it is based on the primary objects of interest rather than their venous drainage.

The anatomy of the middle cerebral artery, by virtue of relative

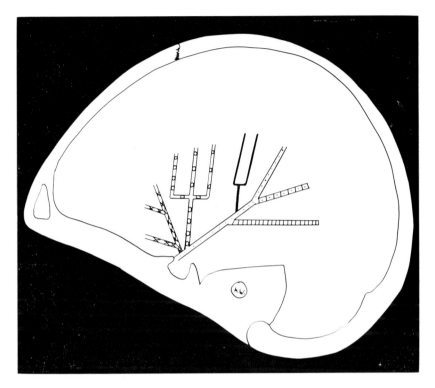

16. SCHEMATIC COURSE OF MIDDLE CEREBRAL ARTERY BRANCHES

This drawing shows the course of the distal branches of the middle cerebral artery. The orbitofrontal branches have a distinct anterior inclination, the operculofrontal branches, after coming out from under the operculum, pass almost directly upward while the central sulcus artery has a slight posterior inclination.

The posterior parietal and angular arteries in their relationship to the axis of the Sylvian fissure suggest an asymmetrical tilted Y, the base of the Y being the axis of the fissure, the upper arm with appreciable upward inclination the posterior parietal, the lower arm with minimal downward inclination being the angular. The posterior temporal branch runs in the long axis of the skull or with a downward inclination.

fixation by the operculum of the insula and the Sylvian fissure, is especially adaptable to outlining zones for the termination of the major branches. The requirements for outlining these areas on the lateral carotid angiogram are that the films used show complete arterial filling with good detail and positioning, as the landmarks are distorted with rotation, and absence of undue magnification. This means that either the head must be positioned in close approximation to the lateral film changer or that a very long target film distance be employed. In general films taken with the head positioned for biplane projections will show appreciable magnification and the absolute figures given may not be suitable. While optimum results require optimum films, the geometry of the template, being based on the midpoint of a variable line, is such as to lessen the errors of magnification and rotation and it is not entirely useless even if films are not perfect. With suitable films, the zones can be outlined as follows:

First, a line is drawn one inch (2.5 cm) from the inner table of the skull, parallel to it, from the roof of the orbits to the internal occipital proturberance. The next line, and most important, is drawn up the axis on the Sylvian vessels to the curved line. In adults with average sized heads, the Taveras clinoparietal line, formed by measuring upward 9 cm from the internal occipital protuberance at right angles to the long axis of the skull and connecting the 9 cm point with a line from the anterior clinoids, can be used. This avoids observer variation in estimating the axis of the Sylvian vessels but is not suitable in children or in patients with excessively large heads, in which cases the axis of the Sylvian vessels must be used. The next step is to bisect the line from the anterior clinoids to the curved line—this midpoint is the key to the entire template. It corresponds closely, but not exactly, to the Sylvian point. From this point, one line drawn upward and parallel to the course of the coronal suture outlines the posterior parietal area behind and the entire ascending frontal complex in front. Another line from the midpoint posteriorly, parallel to a line from the anterior clinoids to the position corresponding to the internal occipital protuberance on the curved line, outlines the angular area superiorly and the temporal area inferiorly.

The ascending frontal area can also be subdivided into three components. By drawing a line anteriorly one inch (2.5 cm) across the tops of the loops of the arteries enfolded in the insula and connecting this with a line drawn upward parallel to the line outlining the posterior parietal area, the position of the motor and sensory strip encompassing the central sulcus and its artery is outlined. The operculofrontal and orbitofrontal arteries, although artificial lines are of less importance in separating them, can be roughly divided by bisecting the remaining

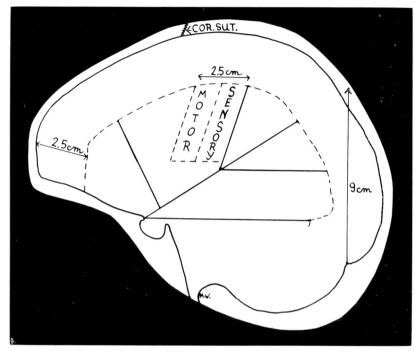

17. TEMPLATE OF AREA SUPPLIED BY BRANCHES OF THE
MIDDLE CEREBRAL ARTERY

The mechanics of forming the template are described in the text. This can
be applied to a plain skull film except for one dimension, this being the dotted
line outlining the lower margin of the motor and sensory strip. This is formed
by drawing a line along the loops of the arteries enfolded under the operculum.

anterior portion of the curved line and connecting this point with a
line up from the dorsum sella.

Although the description of the template is complex the actual
finished product is not. It will seem less complicated and much more
reasonable if one thinks in terms of the fact that the vessels at the end
of the Sylvian fissure must of necessity leave the fissure and pass in
various directions to reach their areas of distribution. The key point
in the template approximates the point where the vessels diverge and
the lines merely fan out from this point in the same way as the vessels.

This template outlines six areas and the respective vessels will be
found to terminate in these areas with a high degree of consistency.
The areas, however, must not be considered to be exact and a slight

overlap of vessels into adjoining zones may be found in normal cases. The one-inch distance from the inner table does not infer that the branches of the middle cerebral artery stop within this area as obviously they do not. This distance was chosen empirically because the branches do attain their individuality proximal to this line and beyond it the terminal twigs of the middle cerebral begin to overlap with similar branches of arteries that have come over the convexity from the midline vessels.

The original template, which has subsequently been somewhat modified, outlined four zones and was devised purely by trial and error, but the reason it is effective is that it is anatomical as shown in the illustration.

Since drawing templates is a slow and laborious task, it is unlikely that this system can be generally used in routine angiography and its use is not essential for the diagnosis of small branch occlusions. The primary benefit obtainable from the template is in calling attention to normal anatomy and it does not take the place of anatomical study. One can apply the principles of zonal arterial distribution without drawing any lines by detailed study of the arterial branches in normal cases. The template helps in becoming familiar with the normal vascular patterns but is an aid and never a substitute for knowledge of anatomy.

The easiest way to identify the branches of the middle cerebral artery on inspection is to start at the bottom, posteriorly, and, with the film facing to the left, go in a counterclockwise manner. The posterior temporal is frequently characteristic in appearance and once this is identified, the angular, posterior parietal and other arteries fall into place like parts of a puzzle. Some experience with normal cases is essential to separate the major from the accessory branches and there is a short cut that can be called the "three finger template" that helps in checking the identify of the arteries by establishing another point of reference. This is done by putting one finger over the sella, one an estimated inch from the inner table of the skull on the axis of the Sylvian vessels, and the middle finger half way between the two. The central sulcus artery will come off either under or just above the middle finger and, using this vessel as a landmark, the adjoining arteries are easily identified.

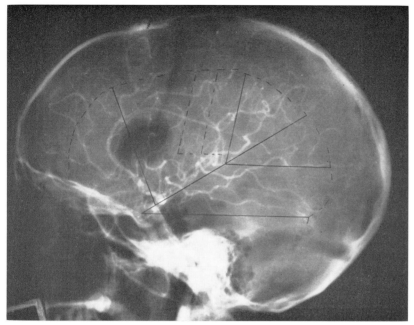

18A. Identification, Frontal Projection

18. IDENTIFICATION OF MIDDLE CEREBRAL ARTERY BRANCHES ON THE FRONTAL PROJECTION

The branches of the middle cerebral artery can usually be distinguished on the frontal projection provided there is good detail and proper angulation. Anatomical detail is best seen in the Chamberlain-Towne (half axial) projection since the x-ray beam is nearly at right angles to the axis of the vessels in the Sylvian fissure. This normal study was done following pneumoencephalography. On the lateral projection (A), the template of the middle cerebral artery is superimposed on the film. The fairly typical candelabra appearance of the operculofrontal branch is accentuated by air in the anterior horns. The frontal projection (B), taken at 30° angulation from Reid's base line, shows the branches well separated for easy identification. These are shown in the drawings identified by various shadings (C and D). The central sulcus artery runs deep in the fissure and is projected more medially than if it were superficial and consequently is well seen as the first major branch directed medially (*solid block*). The posterior parietal is superior, also with some medial inclination. The angular artery, since it reaches the surface with the end of the Sylvian fissure, appears to run laterally before continuing posteriorly. The temporal arteries are inferior and are projected as though they were running medial to the angular.

In young individuals with smooth calvaria and supple spines allowing flexion of the neck, the frontal film should show as much detail as the lateral. Unfortunately, in older individuals in whom the skull is sclerotic or of irregular density and whose dorsal kyphosis make it difficult to get proper angulation, this is sometimes impossible.

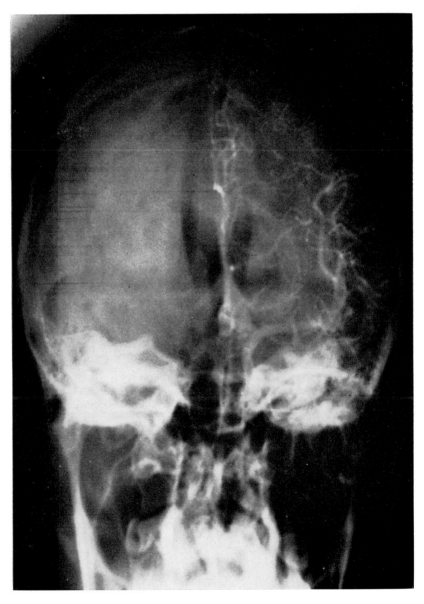

18B. IDENTIFICATION, FRONTAL PROJECTION.
See legend, page 59.

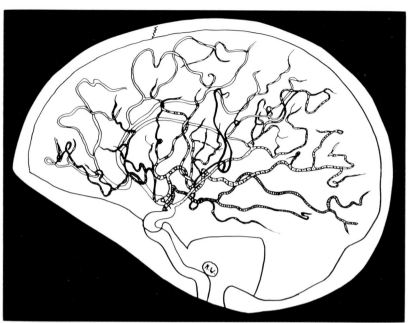

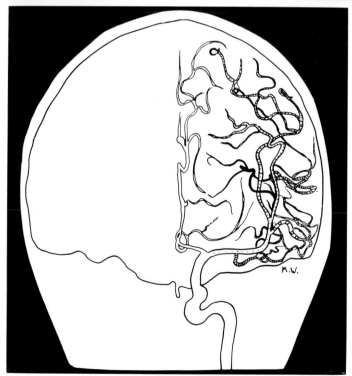

IDENTIFICATION, FRONTAL PROJECTION.
18C. (*Upper*), 18D (*Lower*). See legend, page 59.

——

�→

19. THE THREE FINGER TEMPLATE

With the film facing left, it is more convenient to use the left hand. The axis of the Sylvian fissure is estimated, the index finger placed on this axis an estimated inch from the inner table and the ring finger put over the sella. The middle finger goes on the axis of the vessels half way between the two. The central sulcus artery originates under or in the immediate vicinity of the middle finger.

Occasionally, the central sulcus artery enters the fissure above rather than at the level of the operculum. In such cases, the middle finger approximates the position of the central sulcus and the artery will be seen entering it a little further up. The drawing of the middle cerebral artery branches serves to emphasize the fact that the vessel emerging from under the middle finger actually is the artery to the central sulcus.

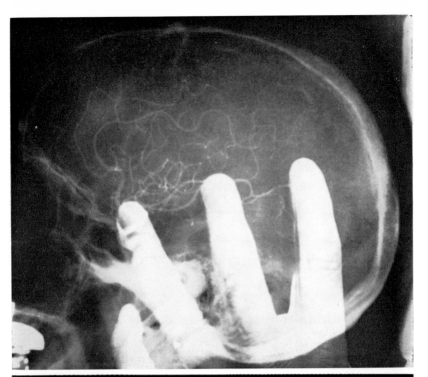

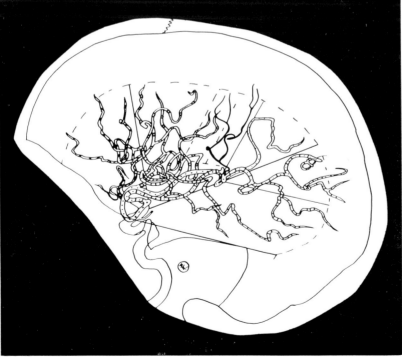

19. THREE FINGER TEMPLATE.
See legend, page 62.

ANTERIOR CEREBRAL AND PERICALLOSAL ARTERIES

THE TERM "anterior cerebral artery" is usually applied to the entire complex of vessels that arise from the carotid and run anteriorly to enter the interhemispheric fissure where they pass around the corpus callosum and continue posteriorly. The portion from the carotid to the anterior communicating artery is the horizontal and that in the interhemispheric fissure, the vertical limbs. Lindgren limits the term, anterior cerebral, to the horizontal limb, the remainder of the complex being the pericallosal vessels. We prefer Lindgren's terminology for two reasons: first, having trained in neuroradiology with Lindgren, we are familiar with this usage, and secondly, these arteries are distinct entities, both angiographically and anatomically so that using two different names is not only justifiable but in our opinion preferable in that it is more specific with less chance of confusion. The same specificity could be obtained by retaining the term, anterior cerebral, and defining the portion under consideration, but anatomical terms of "horizontal limb of the anterior cerebral" and "vertical limb of the anterior cerebral" are a bit cumbersome. Lindgren's terminology is used in the subsequent pages.

The anterior cerebral (the horizontal limb of the anterior cerebral) is not involved in small vessel occlusions and will not be discussed in detail. Occlusions of this artery were described as a cause of cerebrovascular disease by Webster and colleagues but this was on the basis of statistics, the incidence of non-filling of the anterior cerebral considered higher in their patients with cerebrovascular disease than in their controls. We hesitate to diagnose occlusion of this artery without seeing the point of occlusion as it is usually agreed that the artery is very small on one side in some 10% of individuals with both pericallosal groups being supplied by the opposite carotid.

The pericallosal vessels, by our definition, begin at the level of the anterior communicating artery. Although the middle cerebral artery has been considered the most complex and variable of the intracranial vessels, this is actually not the case. The pericallosal arteries appear quite simple on cerebral angiograms as they have a relatively straight course and are sharply silhouetted when filled. They are not end arteries, however, and non-filling when the carotid is well opacified may be due to a small anterior cerebral artery on the injected side or damage to the carotid at the site of puncture so that flow is diminished and both pericallosals supplied by the opposite carotid even when the anterior cerebrals are the same size. Instead of non-filling, there may be partial or incomplete opacification with some contrast containing blood entering from the injected side but being diluted by flow from the contralateral side through the anterior communicating artery. This results in streaming of contrast with non-filling of some normal branches so that a diagnosis of occlusion is impossible. In addition to these problems, true congenital anomalies are common in this location. In brief, these can be divided into three main types. The least frequent is a single, or azygous, pericallosal artery completely supplying both hemispheres that is found in many animals including the rhesus monkey but is extremely rare in the human. However, in about 10% of individuals, one pericallosal artery predominates and supplies most of both hemispheres while its vestigial counterpart supplies only the more anterior portion of the brain on its own side. A third, related to the preceding, and found in some 6 or 7% of individuals, is that of two fairly well developed pericallosal arteries, one of which terminates in the paracentral lobule with the opposing vessel supplying the precuneus on both sides. For details, we recommend Baptista's paper and the interesting case report of LeMay and Gooding. Three pericallosal arteries are occasionally encountered.

To appreciate the anatomy of the pericallosal vessels, it is imperative to see from the frontal projection exactly what vascular arrangements are present. This requires optimum detail and as near a full Towne (half axial) projection as possible. In some cases, bilateral studies with careful correlation of frontal and lateral films are necessary but in the majority there is good filling of one complete pericallosal artery and the areas supplied by the branches can be mapped out on the lateral angiogram much as in the territory of the middle cerebral.

The medial aspect of the cerebral hemisphere is shown in the illus-

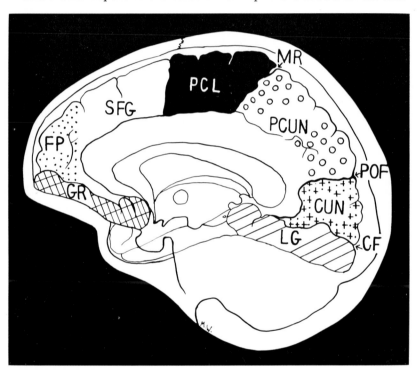

20. MEDIAL ASPECT OF THE CEREBRAL HEMISPHERE. SCHEMATIC
DRAWING WITH AREAS AND LANDMARKS

GR	Gyrus rectus
FP	Frontal Pole
SFG	Superior frontal gyrus
PCL	Paracentral lobule
MR	Marginal Ramus
PCun	Precuneus
POF	Parieto-occipital fissure
Cun	Cuneus
CF	Calcarine fissure
LG	Lingual gyrus

tration with the vascular zones identified with different shadings. The areas may be considered constant although the vessels supplying them are not. Consequently, the use of specific names that are helpful in designating the branches of the middle cerebral artery are likely to cause confusion when applied to branches of the pericallosals. The principle is the same, however—all areas have a constant blood supply irrespective of how it gets there and the first step in appreciating the anatomy of the pericallosal branches is to think first in terms of the brain areas and secondarily of the vessels supplying them. Some terms are so fixed by usage that they must be used and other branches may be accurately named from the areas they supply as long as it is understood that such nomenclature applies only to the case under consideration. The use of the indefinite article helps in making this distinction. It is quite correct to say "there is *a* large frontopolar artery" but stating that "*the* frontopolar artery is large" implies that this vessel is constant and should be seen in all individuals which is not the case.

The branches with generally accepted names are described first since they are familiar to most physicians and will serve as points of reference to the zonal approach.

The parent vessel of the group is the pericallosal itself which typically follows the contour of the corpus callosum and terminates in the area of the precuneus. There is a general misconception that this artery ends in a branch running up the parieto-occipital fissure. This, according to Critchley, is the situation in the baboon but does not apply to the human, the parieto-occipital branch being invariably from the posterior cerebral. Only rarely does the pericallosal artery reach as far posteriorly as the parieto-occipital fissure and its extent in the precuneus varies inversely with the size of branches coming upward from the posterior cerebral. As noted under the discussion of anomalies, it may end without reaching the precuneus in which case the precuneus is supplied by branches from the opposite pericallosal. The relation of the pericallosal artery to the corpus callosum is quite variable and it may run as high as the cingulate sulcus although it never enters the depths of the sulcus. When the pericallosal is high, it often gives off a small branch to the corpus callosum that is clinically important in that its occlusion, with infarction of the corpus callosum, may give rise to bilateral signs.

The callosomarginal artery characteristically arises from the ascending limb of the pericallosal and runs in the cingulate sulcus to terminate in the paracentral lobule. A complete callosomarginal artery, the only one deserving of the name, is present in some 40% of cases, in the majority there are several branches that run for short distances in the cingulate sulcus supplying the same areas.

The frontopolar artery arises from the pericallosal and supplies the frontal pole sending branches around the tip of the frontal pole in the depths of the sulci that may extend laterally for as much as two inches. This artery has been given prominence because of its effect on various types of midline shift but it is only present in about a third of individuals.

Proceeding from the familiar branches to the less familiar concept of areas, those to be considered are the orbital surface of the frontal lobe, the frontal pole, the superior portion of the superior frontal gyrus, the paracentral lobule, precuneus and corpus callosum.

The first area—the medial portion of the orbital surface of the frontal lobe and the gyrus rectus—can be dismissed as an angiographic loser. The vessels in this area are only visible when usually large, as happens in less than 20% and, not rarely, there is crossed circulation to the area from one side to the other. Olfactory groove meningiomas owe some of their angiographic characteristics to these branches since as they are pushed upward they become visible and clearly outline the superior margin of the tumor.

The frontal pole is supplied by the frontopolar artery when it exists —in only one of three cases. In the majority, the area is supplied from more than one source or by recurrent branches coming downward from the superior portion of the superior frontal gyrus. When the orbital branches are unusually large, they extend up and supply the frontal pole, often in conjunction with smaller branches from pericallosal or callosomarginal arteries. Occasionally, there is a cross-circulation to the area from the opposing hemisphere as seen in the orbital area.

The blood supply to the superior portion of the superior frontal gyrus is also variable. At times, there is a large branch going directly to the area that also supplies all or part of the frontal pole. Conversely, when the frontopolar artery is large, it returns the compliment by sending branches upward to the area. The supplying vessel usually comes from the callosomarginal artery when this is present and in cases with unusually large orbitofrontal branches of the middle cerebral there may be a supplementary supply from the lateral aspect of the hemisphere.

There is a good deal of overlap of supplying vessels to these three areas and in the inferior two, at least, the possibilities of a blood supply from the opposite hemisphere in the absence of gross anomalies make the significance of avascular zones less definite than in other areas. It seems fair to say that detecting vascular occlusion by absence of vessels is impossible in the orbital area, difficult in the frontopolar area and not easy in the superior portion of the superior frontal gyrus. These areas are also relatively silent clinically and the conjugate deviation of the eyes associated with infarctions involving the superior portion of the superior frontal gyrus are transient and may not be documented even when occurring so it is rare that clinical correlation with suspected occlusions is possible in these areas.

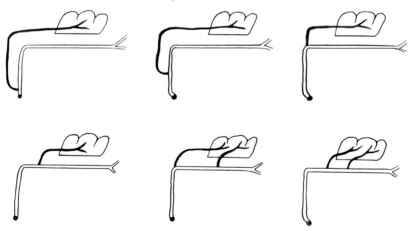

21. SCHEMATIC DRAWING OF THE BLOOD SUPPLY OF THE PARACENTRAL LOBULE

The upper three figures represent variations in the origin of the callosomarginal artery and make up 40% of cases. The branches in the lower tier often run in the cingulate sulcus for short distances but in our opinion do not warrant a specific name other than paracentral branches. In all cases, whether there are one or two supplying arteries, one always enters the area from in front. (Reprinted by permission of *The Amer. J. Roentgenol. Rad. Ther. & Nucl. Med.*)

The paracentral lobule, by contrast, is a bright spot for the anatomist and angiographer. The blood supply to this area is relatively constant, easy to see, and not involved with blood supply from the opposite side except in the presence of anomalies that are obvious on the frontal projection. The term "paracentral branch" has been used to designate the supplying vessel.

For angiographic purposes, the paracentral lobule may be assumed to begin at the level of the coronal suture and extend back to the marginal ramus which can be satisfactorily approximated as being at the level of the line used to separate posterior parietal and central sulcus areas. When the callosomarginal artery exists (40%), it furnishes the blood supply to the area. In about the same number, there is a single large branch from the pericallosal arising just in front of the area that simulates the callosomarginal in all respects except length. In the remaining 20%, there are two good sized arteries, one of which always enters the area from in front.

In the presence of anomalies, both paracentral lobules may be supplied by one artery but we have never encountered a condition in which the blood supply of the paracentral lobule was a combination of vessels from two opposing sides. The blood supply of this area, unlike most of the structures in the interhemispheric fissure, seem to follow the all-or-none law.

The medial portion of the motor strip makes up the medial portion of the paracentral lobule and is involved with leg movements. Occlusions in this area characteristically give rise to a hemiparesis that is most marked in the leg, so good clinical correlation is possible.

The precuneus, behind the paracentral lobule, varies considerably in size, unlike the paracentral lobule which is fairly constant, and has a variable blood supply, this being a combination of the pericallosal artery and the posterior cerebral in the majority of cases with cross circulation from the opposing pericallosal in some 6 to 7%.

The marginal ramus, separating the paracentral lobule and the precuneus, is outlined by an artery in about 60% of cases that is usually a branch of the pericallosal. Occasionally, the callosomarginal artery or branches simulating it terminate in the marginal ramus but never cross it. In addition to the use of the template, the marginal ramus may be located by its relationship with the central sulcus artery. If the axis of the central sulcus is extended upward, the marginal ramus reaches the convexity a centimeter or so behind it. Vessels with an identical course may be found both in front and behind this point, so it is not an obvious landmark.

POSTERIOR CEREBRAL ARTERIES

THE POSTERIOR CEREBRAL ARTERIES are difficult to study angiographically due to the frequency with which streaming and incomplete filling occur. Omitting the penetrating vessels, there are two main divisions—occipital and temporal (medial and lateral)—that outline the lingual gyrus between them. The temporal branch supplies the inferior aspect of the temporal lobe, the occipital branch, the occipital lobe. Both of these major trunks divide, the division of the temporal artery being somewhat variable while the division of the occipital artery into calcarine and parieto-occipital branches is quite constant. The occipital branch divides at the junction of the parieto-occipital and calcarine fissure sending a small branch up the calcarine fissure while the larger component goes up the parieto-occipital fissure. In about 80% of cases, branches from the artery in the parieto-occipito fissure extend into the precuneus and as previously noted vary inversely in size with branches to the same area from the pericallosal. These branches tend to run in the depths of the fissure rather than on the surface of the medial aspect of the hemisphere so that on the frontal projection of angiograms they are located laterally to the midline.

In our very limited experience with isolated occlusion of one of the two major branches of the posterior cerebral artery, diagnosed by vertebral angiography, retrograde filling of the occluded component by collateral flow has not been prominent. We have seen more examples of posterior cerebral occlusion on carotid angiograms that

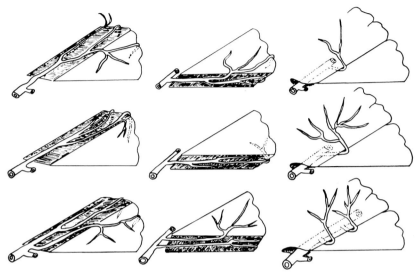

PARIETO-OCCIPITAL ART.　　CALCARINE ART.(ies)　　PRECUNEAL ART.(ies).

22. PATTERNS OF THE PARIETO-OCCIPITAL, CALCARINE AND PRE-
CUNEAL BRANCHES OF THE POSTERIOR CEREBRAL ARTERY

These schematic drawings are made from the medial aspect of the hemisphere
and slightly obliqued to show the depths of the fissures. The branches of the
artery in the parieto-occipital fissure, shown with three common arrangements
on the left, run predominantly downward over both the medial and posterior
aspects of the cuneus of the occipital lobe. The distal branches of the artery
in the calcarine fissure run upward, either medially or posteriorly, to supply
the same area. The branches to the precuneus arise from the parieto-occipital
branch and leave the fissure on the medial aspect of the hemisphere to run
upward and anteriorly. The extent of these latter vessels vary inversely with
those coming posteriorly from the pericallosal artery.

were diagnosed by the occurrence of retrograde collateral filling but
in these cases it is often impossible to be sure whether or not the entire
posterior cerebral is involved. It is not difficult to recognize occlusion
of the main trunks of the posterior cerebral if this is well opacified
on vertebral angiograms as there are only two major branches that
have a divergent course on the frontal projection and from inspection
one can readily tell whether they are present or absent. Since the
temporal branch may arise separately from the basilar, its absence on
a carotid study with opacification of the posterior cerebral may not
be due to occlusion. Occlusions of the posterior cerebral artery as a
whole were discussed by Mones and colleagues in 1961.

The Neglected Cause of Stroke

The zones of the arterial supply of pericallosal and posterior cerebral arteries do not lend themselves to delineation in such a neat template as that applied to the branches of the middle cerebral artery, but artificial landmarks can be used to some extent and are helpful. The paracentral lobule shows very little variation in length and its anterior

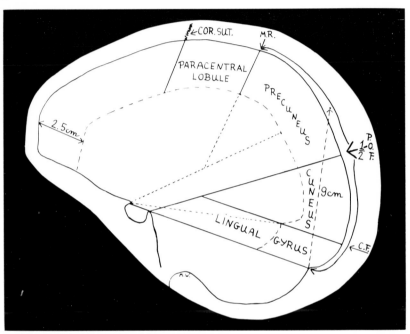

23. TEMPLATE FOR THE AREAS SUPPLIED BY PERICALLOSAL AND POSTERIOR CEREBRAL ARTERIES

By starting with the template used for branches of the middle cerebral artery (*dotted lines*), the position of the marginal ramus can be approximated by extending the line separating central sulcus and posterior parietal areas to the inner table of the skull. The para-central lobule lies in front of this line and can be assumed to begin at the level of the coronal suture. Posteriorly, the precuneus can be assumed to occupy half the distance from the marginal ramus (M.R.) to the internal occipital protuberance. The lingual gyrus can be approximated as the area between the two solid lines, the lowermost going from the internal occipital protuberance to the tuberculum sella, the one above being parallel to it and running through the point corresponding to the internal occipital protuberance on the curved line. This upper line roughly corresponds to the calcarine fissure (C.F.), and the cuneus lies above it.

Although drawing in the areas of the lingual gyrus may require more work than the information gained is worth, the approximate position of the parieto-occipital fissure can be determined without undue difficulty and is a valuable landmark.

limits can be approximated as being at the level of the coronal suture. The termination of the paracentral lobule at the marginal ramus can, as previously described, be assumed to be opposite the line separating the posterior parietal and central sulcus areas on the template applied to the branches of the middle cerebral. The precuneus, as opposed to the paracentral lobule, is quite variable in length. Waddington, in adult brains, found this variation to be up to 100%. There seems to be relation with skull shape and perhaps the pronounced variability in length of the precuneus compensates for the relatively constant length of the paracentral lobule in the diverse contours of the cranial vault. To separate precuneus and cuneus, Waddington suggested merely halving the distance along the outer table of the skull from the marginal ramus as estimated from the extension of the line between posterior parietal and central sulcus arteries to the occipital protuberance. This has given satisfactory results when applied to carotid angiograms in which the posterior cerebral artery is filled sufficiently to opacify the artery in the parieto-occipital fissure. Since these landmarks are based on alignment of lateral and medial structures, they are particularly susceptible to distortion by rotation and true lateral projections are essential for their use. Detailed directions for forming a template for this area are given with the illustration.

SECTION 13

NORMAL ANATOMY AND POST MORTEM CORRELATION

The following section is purely illustrative and is included to show examples of the anatomical detail previously described. The first series of illustrations are a case on which angiographic details were correlated with post mortem dissection of the cerebral arteries. The second series is a group of drawings of vessels dissected from normal post mortem brain specimens, that were selected from a large series prepared by Dr. Waddington, to show examples of the commonly encountered variations. Angiograms and drawing of a normal vertebral study are included for completeness, although the vertebrobasilar system is not discussed in any depth. Perhaps most important are the group of cases showing post mortem correlation of infarcts with the angiographic findings of occlusions. The two cases of normal variants simulating occlusion as compared to an occlusion giving a very similar appearance may serve as a warning that the diagnosis of branch occlusion must be based on anatomical facts and can seldom be made by superficial inspection.

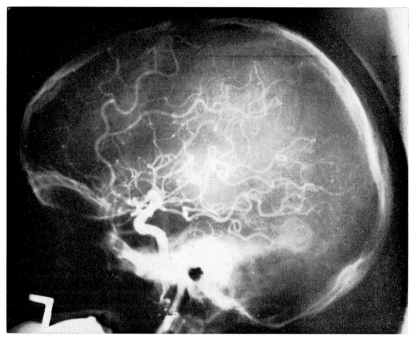

24A.

24. NORMAL ANATOMY

Normal studies showing all three major supratentorial arteries in whom post mortem dissection of vessels are possible are rarely encountered. The patient illustrated here (A) had no brain abnormality and died shortly after the study from an unrelated cause.

The relationship of the middle cerebral branches to the template is shown in the first drawing (B). The topography of the lateral surface of the hemisphere is shown in the next drawing (C) with the sulci dotted in and the temporal pole, motor and sensory strip and the angular gyrus darkened by stippling to serve as reference points.

The vessels of the medial aspect of the hemisphere are shown in drawing (D) with the landmarks outlining the paracentral lobule and marginal ramus in solid lines and the template for the branches of the posterior cerebral artery drawn in. The last drawing shows the structures of the medial aspect of the hemisphere dotted in with the paracentral lobule and cuneus identified by stippling.

The purpose of these sketches is to emphasize that cerebral angiograms are not a haphazard arrangement of white streaks on a darker background but a surprisingly precise display of living anatomy. The arteries may show some variation, but in the end their entire arrangement is based on the relationships of anatomical structures. If one develops the habit of thinking in terms of these areas when studying angiograms, previously undetected abnormalities become obvious and the normal variation in course and manner of division of the arteries of no significance.

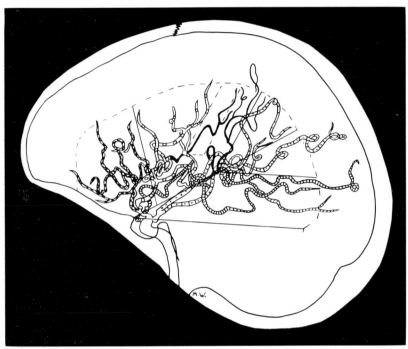

See legend, page 77.

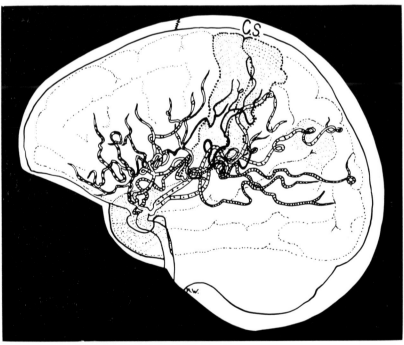

24B (*Upper*), 24C (*Lower*). See legend, page 77.

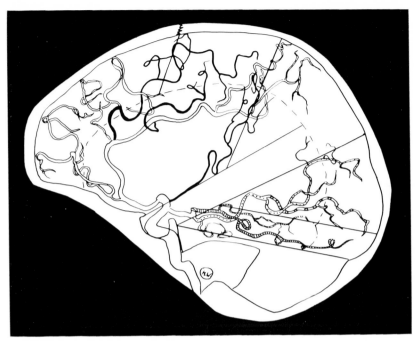

24D. See legend, page 77.

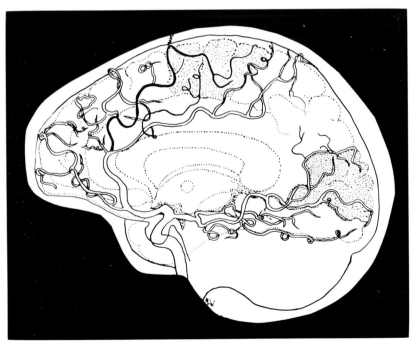

24D (*Upper*), 24E (*Lower*). See legend, page 77.

25. NORMAL ANATOMY: DRAWING OF VESSELS DISSECTED AT POST MORTEM

Much of the confusing appearance of the arteries on cerebral angiograms is due to their three dimensional course which results in considerable overlap. With the vessels straightened out after removal from the depths of the sulci, they are little more complex than arteries elsewhere.

The following representative cases are taken from drawings made of post mortem vessel dissections. It is hoped that they will help convince the viewer that the intracranial arteries do in fact have a constant distribution and that the apparently endless variations are primarily in the course and manner of division of the branches, modified to some extent by the inverse size relationship that is always present when two branches from different sources supply contiguous areas.

In the following illustrations, the branches to the central sulcus, the paracentral lobule and the branches from the posterior cerebral artery to the precuneus are in solid black. The branches of the middle and posterior cerebral arteries are identified with the same type of shading as is used throughout the book. The pericallosal and posterior cerebral arteries are shown together on one figure, with the middle cerebral artery branches on the following illustration. The abbreviations, POF and CF are for parieto-occipital fissure and calcarine fissure.

Case 1 A. The orbital arteries are large and give rise to a frontopolar branch. The paracentral lobule is supplied by a callosomarginal artery that arises at the knee of the pericallosal. The precuneus is supplied entirely by the pericallosal artery and no branches reach this area from the posterior cerebral. The remainder of the posterior cerebral artery is not remarkable except for rather large anterior temporal arteries. (The anterior temporal branches of both the middle and posterior cerebral arteries are usually ignored on angiograms as they are ordinarily poorly seen.)

B. The middle cerebral branches arise separately near the mouth of fissure, a condition better appreciated on dissections since on angiograms the trunks are superimposed in the Sylvian fissure. The ascending frontal complex arises as a unit and the orbitofrontal branches are small in keeping with the large orbital branches of the pericallosal. The other branches are nearly of equal size.

Case 2 A. The orbital vessels are small, the paracentral lobule supplied by one large branch from the pericallosal which terminates with only minor twigs to the precuneus. The precuneal branches from the parieto-occipital branch of the posterior cerebral are very large. Note the prominent lateral branches of the posterior cerebral that are probably compensatory for the rather puny posterior temporal branches of the middle.

B. The orbito-frontal vessels are large and share one trunk with the operculofrontal which has an arrangement not in the least resembling a candelabrum. There are two central sulcus arteries and a posterior branch of the operculofrontal serves as an accessory blood supply to the motor strip. The central sulcus arteries arise from a branch that terminates as an accessory posterior parietal. The posterior parietal proper, the angular and a posterior temporal branch all arise from one trunk.

Case 3 A. The orbital and frontopolar branches are small, the paracentral lobule supplied by two branches from the pericallosal. The pericallosal sends a prominent branch up the marginal ramus and terminates in the precuneus, sharing the blood supply of this area with the branches from the posterior cerebral. Note the small branch continuing from the pericallosal artery that is commonly present and supplies the corpus callosum when the pericallosal artery has a high course in the inter-hemispheric fissure. There are two branches from the posterior cerebral in the calcarine fissure and the anterior temporal branch is very small.

B. The small anterior temporal branch of the posterior cerebral is compensated by the very large anterior temporal branch of the middle, this being shown as the most inferior of the arteries directed posteriorly. The orbitofrontal branches are enormous and arise as two separate branches. The operculo-frontal and one central sulcus artery share a common trunk of origin, while a second artery to the central sulcus arises from the posterior parietal. All vessels have their origin proximally in the Sylvian fissure and the posterior temporal artery arises as two separate branches.

Case 4 A. There is a typical callosomarginal artery supplying the paracentral lobule and the blood supply to the precuneus is shared between pericallosal and posterior cerebral branches. The lateral branch of the posterior cerebral arises as two distinct arteries and the anterior temporal branch is small.

B. In this individual, the three components of the ascending frontal branch have separate origins. There is a prominent trifurcation of the operculofrontal branch, one central sulcus artery and an accessory posterior parietal artery. The anterior temporal is very large, approximating the size of the posterior temporal.

Case 5 A. There is a very large frontopolar branch that supplies the frontal lobe up as far as the paracentral lobule. The pericallosal has abundant branching in the precuneus and no vessels to the area are found from the posterior cerebral. The lateral branch of the posterior cerebral arises proximally and also serves as the anterior temporal component.

B. Two orbitofrontal branches arise individually, while the operculofrontal and two central sulcus arteries share one trunk. There is a prominent candelabrum-like arrangement of the operculofrontal. The three posterior branches arise distally from one large trunk, a condition pleasing to see angiographically since with this arrangement the individual vessels are seen without superimposition and are very easy to identify. A moderately prominent anterior temporal artery compensates for the distal origin of the posterior temporal.

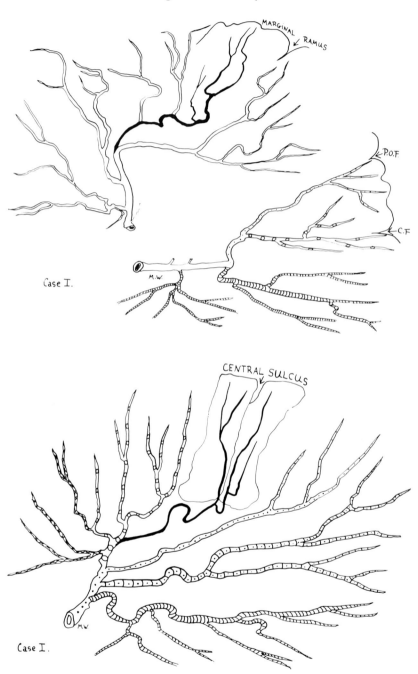

25A. (*Upper*), 25B (*Lower*). See legend, page 80.

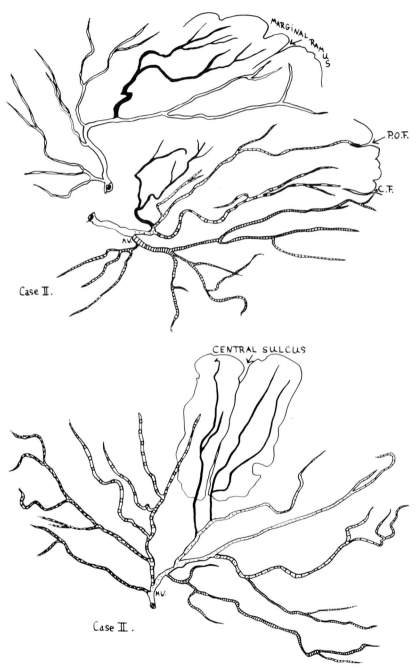

Case II.

Case II.

25A (*Upper*), 25B (*Lower*). See legend, page 80.

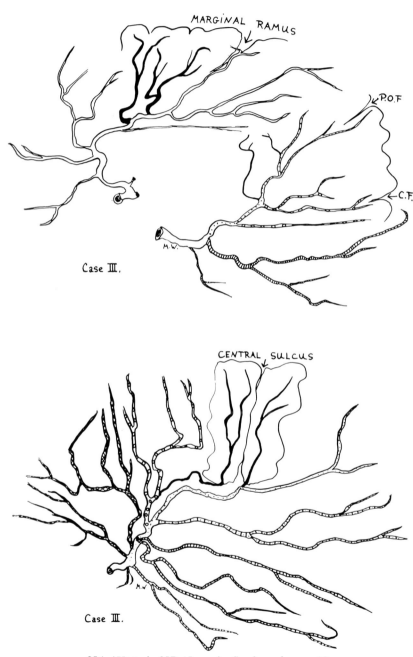

MARGINAL RAMUS

P.O.F

C.F.

M.W.

Case III.

CENTRAL SULCUS

M.W.

Case III.

25A (*Upper*), 25B (*Lower*). See legend, page 80.

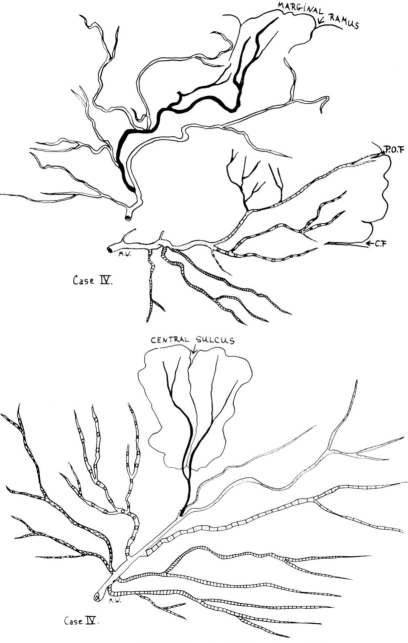

Case IV.

Case IV.

25A (*Upper*), 25B (*Lower*). See legend, page 80.

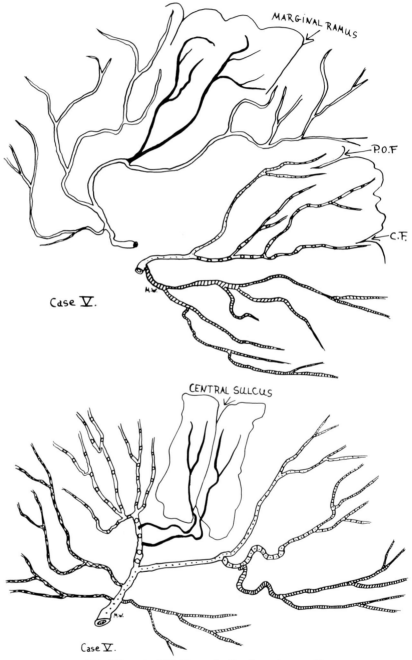

Case V.

Case V.

25A (*Upper*), 25B (*Lower*). See legend, page 80.

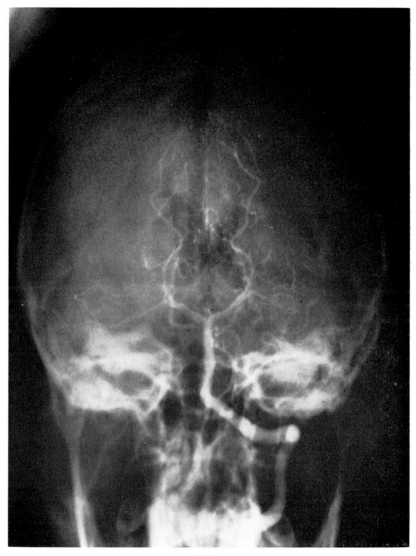

26A.

26. NORMAL VERTEBRAL ANGIOGRAM

The anatomy of the infratentorial arteries is worthy of more attention than can be given here. This normal study is included for two reasons: (1) For a better look at the posterior cerebral artery since, when this is filled from the carotid, there is some superimposition on both frontal and lateral and, (2) because one abnormal vertebral study is included.

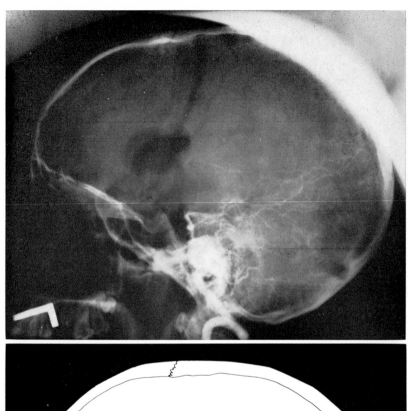

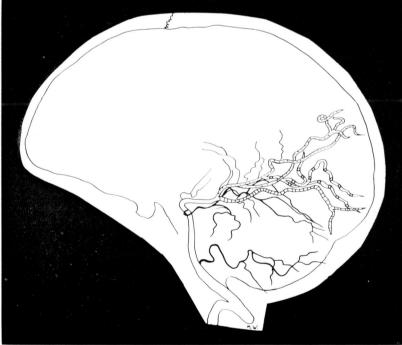

26B (*Upper*), 26C (*Lower*). See legend, page 87.

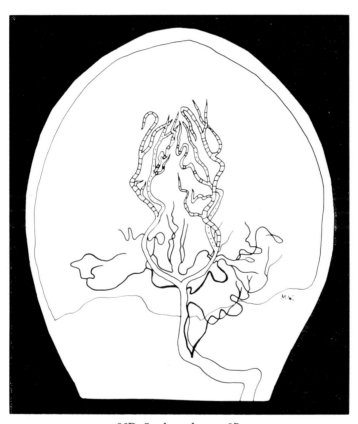

26D. See legend, page 87.

The Neglected Cause of Stroke

27. POST MORTEM CORRELATION WITH OCCLUSIONS
DIAGNOSED BY ANGIOGRAPHY

It is seldom possible to confirm angiographic findings of an isolated branch occlusion at post mortem as patients ordinarily do not die of the single episode. If the isolated occlusion merely heralds a progressive and fatal process, such as generalized embolization, its identity is lost in the presence of the numerous occlusions and massive infarction responsible for death. Since post mortem correlation was possible in one case in which the patient died without further central nervous system involvement, it is worth discussing in detail.

The patient, whose films are presented, was an elderly lady who had resided in a nursing home since a stroke, clinically diagnosed as thrombosis of the right middle cerebral artery, one year previously. She was partially ambulatory despite the left hemiparesis and one evening was found unconscious after a fall. An angiogram was requested because of a possible subdural hematoma and the left side done in view of the probable occlusion of the middle cerebral on the right. There was no evidence of subdural, but there was an abrupt occlusion of the posterior parietal branch of the middle cerebral visible both on frontal and lateral projections. The patient was treated symptomatically, but did not improve, went into pulmonary edema and died three days later. At post mortem, the cerebral vessels were dissected free, photographed and drawn, and are seen for correlation with the angiogram.

The first figure is the lateral angiogram (A). The background of fine lines is artefactual and due to cracks in the emulsion of the film from accidental overheating. There is a prominent external vessel over the posterior parietal area but the posterior parietal artery itself is absent.

The details of angiographic anatomy are better seen on the drawing (B) than on the radiograph since the confusing superficial and meningeal vessels are omitted. There is a small accessory posterior parietal artery behind two central sulcus arteries and these are bowed slightly anteriorly from edema in the area of infarction. There is a prominent frontopolar branch of the pericallosal artery and all vessels show moderate changes of arteriosclerosis.

On the frontal projections, both film and drawing (C and D) show the point of occlusion of the posterior parietal branch to good advantage.

The pericallosal artery, dissected free, is shown as photographed (E) and drawn (F). The blood supply of the paracentral lobule is in solid black. The vessels are strikingly similar to the appearance on the angiogram. The middle cerebral artery branches are shown in G and H. In the photograph of the middle cerebral artery (G), the central sulcus arteries are identified by black squares and the occlusions by arrows. In the drawing, the arteries are identified by shading, the points of occlusion emphasized by arrows. There was found to be an additional occlusion of a small posterior branch of the posterior of two central sulcus arteries.

The cut surface of the brain (I) is an anterior-posterior projection so the left side is on the viewer's left, reversed from the customary orientation of angiograms. The old infarct, deep, just under the cortex of the operculum is quite obvious on the right. On the left the predominantly cortical infarct is seen just above the Sylvian fissure. Some of the necrotic cortical tissue was lost in sectioning the brain.

The correlation between angiogram and dissected vessels prove the reliability of the angiogram in accurately portraying vascular anatomy.

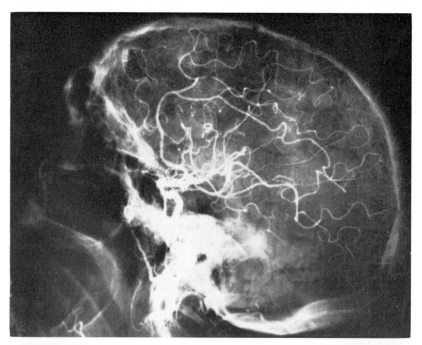

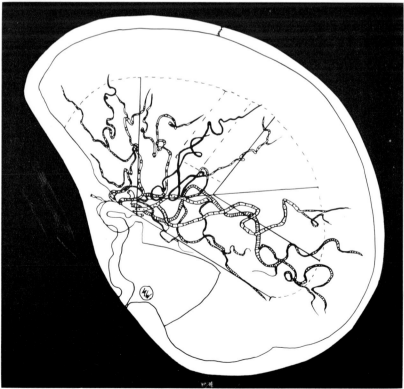

27A (*Upper*), 27B (*Lower*). See legend, page 90.

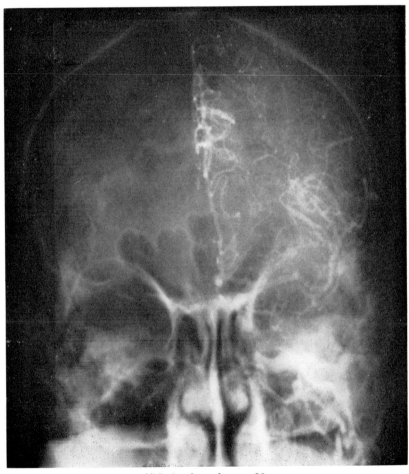

27C. See legend, page 90.

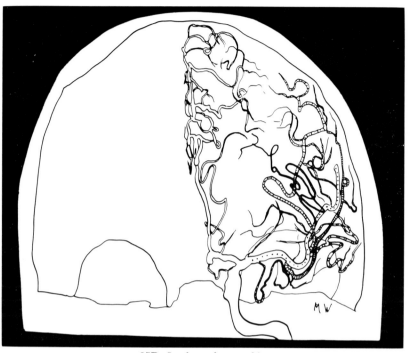

27D. See legend, page 90.

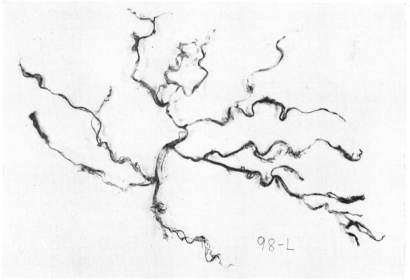

27E. See legend, page 90.

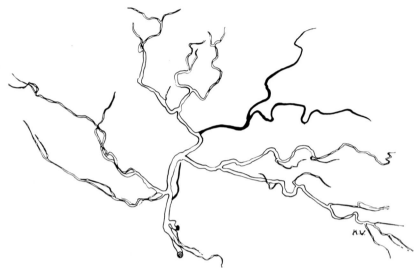

27F. See legend, page 90.

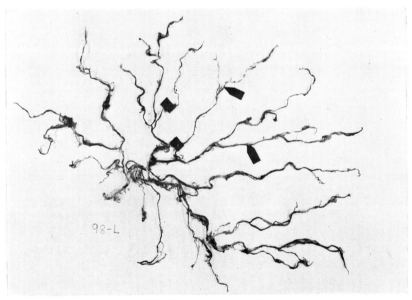

27G. See legend, page 90.

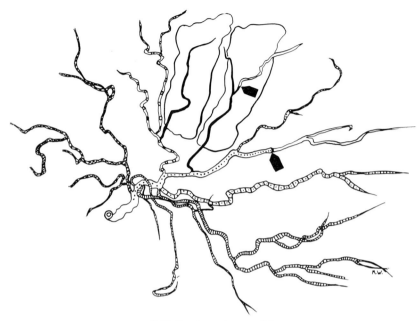

27H. See legend, page 90.

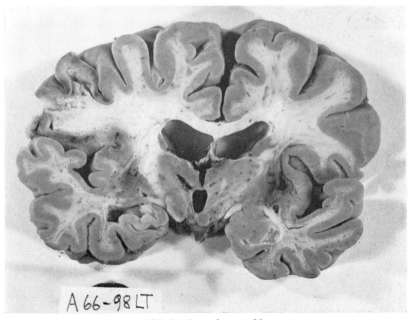

27I. See legend, page 90.

The Neglected Cause of Stroke

28. POST MORTEM CORRELATION WITH OCCLUSION OF PERICALLOSAL ARTERY

The following case was supplied by Doctor Waddington with the cooperation of the Radiology (Doctor Sherban) and Pathology (Doctor Stowens) Departments of St. Lukes Hospital, Utica, New York.

The patient was a 68-year-old hypertensive diabetic with an organic brain syndrome who developed sudden right leg paresis. Angiography was done to exclude an underlying tumor with the findings shown in the illustrations. The patient's course was progressively downhill; she developed bilateral neurological signs, became comatose and died three weeks later.

On an early film of the lateral angiograph (A), there is generalized arteriosclerosis of the internal carotid and all intracranial arteries. There is a large pericallosal that gives off branches to the frontal pole, superior frontal gyrus and one branch that extends into the paracentral lobule. Just distal to this branch the pericallosal artery comes to an end. On a later film (B), the dye column in the occluded vessel has progressed only a few millimeters. None of the secondary signs of occlusion were present. The central sulcus artery is included on the drawing (C).

The brain specimen (D) is shown facing to the *right* since the left hemisphere was involved. The paracentral lobule is outlined by a black marker and the thrombus in the pericallosal artery stands out as a black area in the otherwise white vessel. There is some discoloration of the distal portion of the paracentral lobule due to infarction and although it is not apparent on the photograph, the corpus callosum in its posterior part was soft, mushy and completely infarcted.

The dissected vessels (E) are photographed, also facing to the *right*. There are three branches distal to the occlusion, one large branch that bifurcates and supplies the majority of paracentral lobules, another going into the percuneus and bifurcating and a third, the smallest and most inferior, was the supplying artery to the posterior portion of the corpus callosum. This branch, discussed under the anatomy of the pericallosal vessels is inconstant but of considerable practical importance since the bilateral signs associated with its occlusion may suggest a process other than vascular disease.

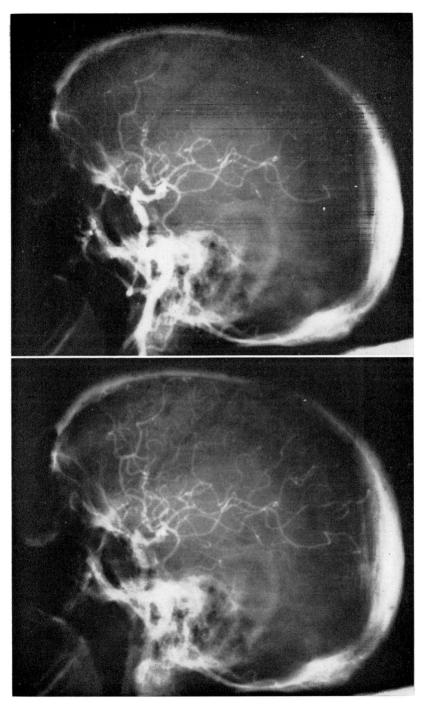

28A (*Upper*), 28B (*Lower*). See legend, page 96.

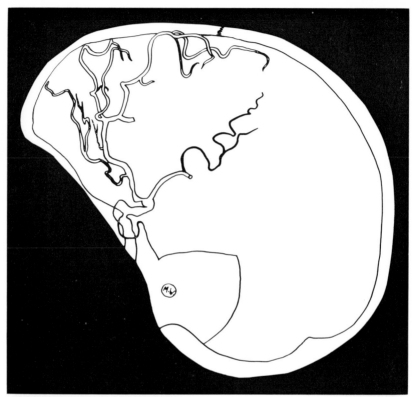

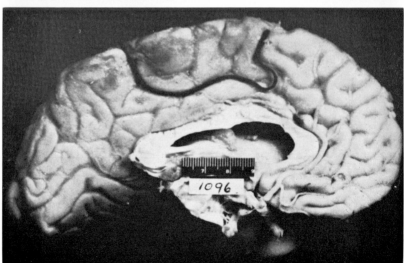

28C (*Upper*), 28D (*Lower*). See legend, page 96.

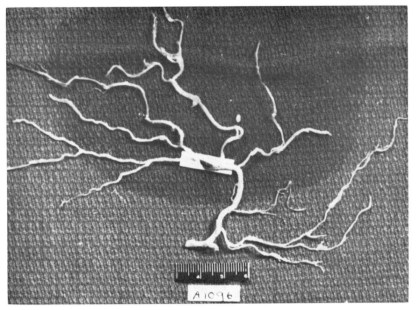

28D. See legend, page 96.

29. NORMAL VARIANT SIMULATING OCCLUSION

Although the areas supplied by the branches of the middle cerebral artery are constant, the vessels may vary considerably in their course to these areas. The first patient (A) was examined after a step-like series of episodes leading to progressive deterioration that was clinically suggestive of multiple small artery occlusions. There are two large arteries at the end of the Sylvian fissure with a wide space between them and it would be tempting to consider this the result of an occlusion. Closer analysis of the vessels, however, show that all are present (B) although the large angular artery has a high course and is in close approximation to the posterior parietal.

A similar condition is seen in the film of the next patient (C). Again, on close analysis, all arteries are present (D) and there is an unusual vessel that appears to be a third artery in the central sulcus area. This individual had no clinical evidence of occlusive vascular disease.

The first patient was subsequently found to have herpes simplex encephalitis and there may be some element of displacement from focal edema, but the basic change is that of a normal variant.

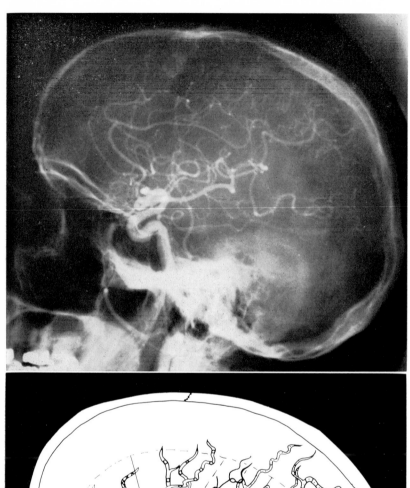

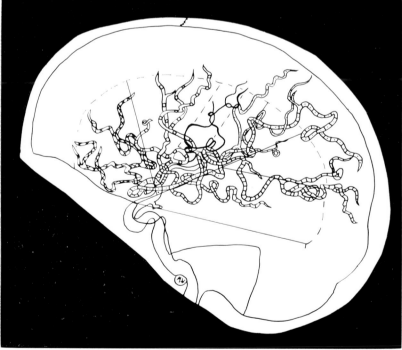

29A (*Upper*), 29B (*Lower*). See legend, page 99.

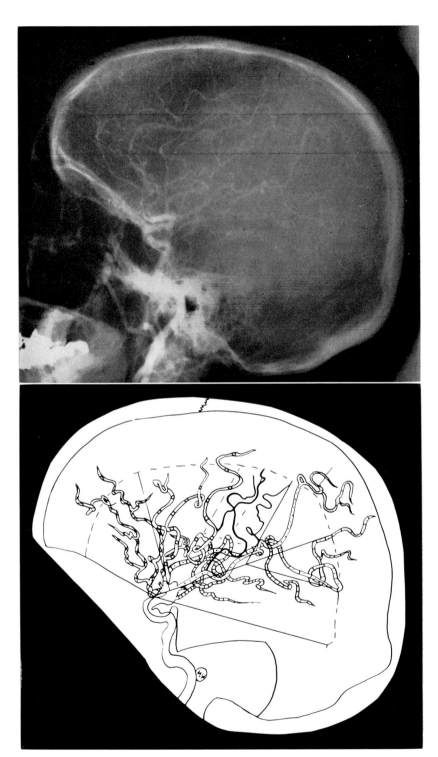

29C (*Upper*), 29D (*Lower*). See legend, page 99.

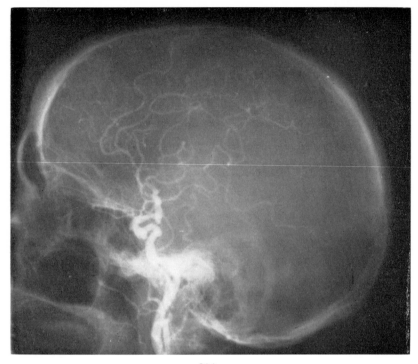

30A.

30. GROSS OCCLUSION RESEMBLING NORMAL VARIANT

On superficial inspection, there is a resemblance between the angiogram of this patient (A) and the two cases presented as normal variants. On a second look, however, there is no similarity whatsoever. The previous two patients had the normal component of vessels with an unusual space between two of them. The avascular space in this patient is due to occlusion.

The patient was a 70-year-old lady with hypertension and polycythemia who developed slowly progressive parietal lobe signs suggesting tumor rather than vascular disease.

On the angiogram there is extensive and generalized intracranial arteriosclerosis with gross changes in the internal carotid. There is a large posterior temporal branch but nothing above it until a large central sulcus artery, with proximal branching, is encountered. The absence of the angular and posterior parietal branches is even more obvious on the drawing (B). The two branches may have shared a common trunk that was occluded proximally. The ascending frontal complex in this individual arises as a single trunk.

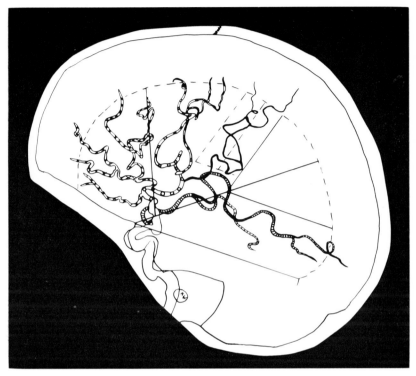

30B. See legend, page 102.

SECTION 14

INTRACRANIAL EMBOLI

A<small>LTHOUGH INTRACRANIAL OCCLUSIONS</small> may be due to a multiplicity of causes, the vast majority represent either primary thrombosis associated with atherosclerosis or emboli. After having been relatively neglected in the radiological literature for years, the embolic occlusion has recently been given more attention. In any discussion of intracranial emboli, two questions must be answered: first, where do they come from and, secondly, what are the angiographic criteria for diagnosis.

So firmly has the heart been intrenched as the number one source of intracranial emboli that nine times out of ten if one tells an internist that cerebral angiography suggests intracranial emboli in the noncardiac patient, the reply will be an automatic denial—"but - he doesn't have atrial fibrillation - (or - valvular disease - or - myocardial infarction.)" In our experience, the heart is a poor third as a source of intracranial emboli. The carotid arteries are first, unknown sources next and a cardiac origin in the minority. The reason for this deviation from time honored medical dogma is, in our opinion, due to the fact that emboli from the heart have usually been recognized as such, while emboli from other sources have not. The thrombi associated with atrial fibrillation or myocardial infarcts give rise to good size fragments that occlude the larger arteries and the underlying disease process and the acute effect of the embolus are obvious, both clinically and in cases coming to post mortem. The vegetations embolizing from an endocarditis may be smaller but are so often associated with typical systemic

[104]

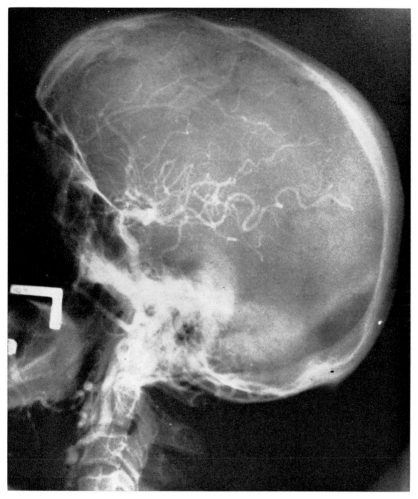

31A.

31. PROPAGATION OF THROMBUS IN THE CAROTID ARTERY

This 55-year-old man was examined a few days after a bout of transient hemiparesis. He was completely asymptomatic at the time of angiography and the only positive finding was a small filling defect in the carotid sinus (first angiogram film). The patient declined surgery so was placed on anti-coagulants. Two months later he was readmitted with a recurrent stroke and a rapidly progressing downhill course. Of particular interest in the second examination is the extension of the thrombus in the carotid sinus that is now filling much of the lumen with irregularities and the undercut upper edge of

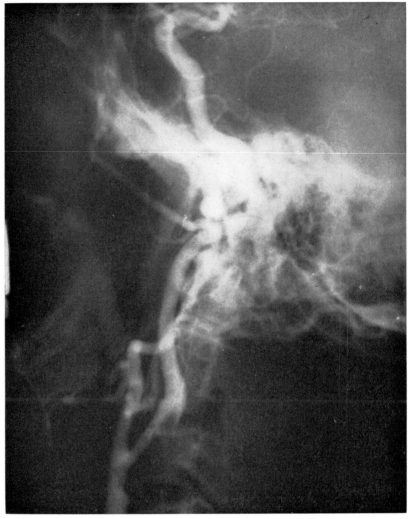

31B. Propagation of Thrombus

the filling defect typical of a propagating thrombus (enlargement). On later films of the intercranial arteries, there were multiple occlusions.

Such massive intra-arterial thrombi are not as common in our experience as the smaller ones, perhaps because patients with the multiple emboli expected under these circumstances do so poorly that angiography is seldom performed. Obviously, anticoagulants were not the answer to this patient's problem and he died with infarction of the entire hemisphere. (Reprinted by courtesy of *Amer. J. Roentgenol., Rad. Ther. & Nucl. Med.*)

manifestations and emboli elsewhere that they too are obvious. Emboli from other sources are frequently not suspected as a cause for stroke and since complete extra- and intracranial vascular dissections are rarely routine post mortem procedures, the smaller noncardiac emboli are seldom documented.

The mural thrombi at the carotid bifurcation that we consider the most common source of intracranial emboli may be large or small, occur in the old or relatively young, and their appearance on angiograms varying from the obvious, with a large filling defect with an undercut upper edge projecting into the lumen of the artery, to minor irregularities that may easily be overlooked. Despite the wide range of possibilities, large series of patients with intracranial emboli do show some definite tendencies. In our experience, the majority occur in a younger age group than primary stenosing lesions, they tend to be restricted to one artery, have little evidence of systemic or intracranial arteriosclerosis and, as Wood noted, in general are smaller than the stenosing lesions. These characteristics suggest that the process is frequently one of the accidental secondary manifestations of rapidly developing atherosclerosis that appears before the vascular tree as a whole undergoes irreversible change. If this assumption is correct, these are the patients who would receive the greatest benefit and return the greatest benefit to society from treatment minimizing the acute episode and preventing recurrence.

There is little to add to the secondary source of intracranial emboli— "unknown." Some arise from ulcerated atheroma in the aorta but this is difficult to prove during life. Other sources are speculative, but ulcerating lesions in or at the origins of the great cerebral vessels proximal to the carotid sinus are possibilities as are paradoxical emboli from systemic sources. The latter cannot be excluded on the absence of pulmonary infarctions as emboli too small to cause pulmonary changes may well be catastrophic in the brain. In addition, mural thrombi in the carotid sinus may exist and escape detection at angiography.

Emboli from the heart are so familiar that they need no further discussion. Dissecting aneurysms of the ascending aorta not infrequently produce emboli to the brain and there is always the possibility of embolization after surgery on the heart or proximal great vessels in the chest. The relationship between the embolism and the under-lying process in these conditions is obvious.

Emboli to the basilar system may be expected to have the same general origins (not necessarily with the same frequency) but are not discussed here as we have had insufficient experience with them to make any worthwhile comments.

Although there are criteria for the angiographic diagnosis of embolic occlusions, they are not absolute. In some cases, the diagnosis is obvious, but frequently it is not. Emboli can and should be suggested as possibilities in many cases that do not fill the criteria if one remembers two facts—first, that embolic occlusions are common and, secondly, that intracranial occlusions do not occur without a reason. In the absence of intracranial arteriosclerosis (or arteritis or systemic disorders), an acute stroke with angiographic changes limited to absence of a single branch is most likely due to an embolus.

The criteria for the diagnosis of embolic occlusions that Lund presented for us in 1965 have been modified by others, primarily from observations on emboli occurring during cerebral angiography. The characteristics commonly found with such iatrogenic emboli have been rare in our series of occlusions and have been found primarily in cases with generalized embolization who were doing badly. The reason for the discrepancies is the time element between embolization and the angiogram. Iatrogenic emboli are seen immediately, whereas ordinarily angiography is not performed for some time after an intracranial occlusion. The similarities between iatrogenic emboli and our experience with patients doing poorly, in whom angiography is done in desperation, is due to the fact that in the latter cases fresh emboli are continually arriving in the cerebral circulation and are seen, as are the iatrogenic ones, before they have stabilized.

Criteria for the angiographic diagnosis of intracranial emboli can be summarized as follows:

(1) Embolic fragments visible in the lumen of the intracranial vessels. (Diagnostic, but rare in clinical cases.)

(2) Multiple occlusions in the absence of intracranial arteriosclerosis or other conditions that may produce vascular occlusion. This should include the secondary signs of occlusion, local delayed circulation time, stasis, etc.

(3) Abrupt, round-edged occlusion in a normal vessel as opposed to the tapering usually associated with arteriosclerosis.

(4) Movement or disappearance of an occlusive process on repeat injection or subsequent angiogram.

(5) Visible or known source of emboli.

32. GENERALIZED INTRACRANIAL EMBOLIZATION FROM KNOWN SOURCE

This case is more helpful as a demonstration of pathology than practical application since the prognosis with such extensive disease is virtually hopeless. The patient had surgery for the subclavian steal syndrome but later thrombosed at the site of the graft and after re-operation developed rapidly progressive neurological changes and became comatose. The study was performed on the chance that a large, single embolus might be located and surgically removed.

On the first radiograph (A), there is evidence of a greatly prolonged circulation time. The intracranial arteries that remain patent are still opacified and there is early filling of the central veins. There are multiple occlusions involving the middle cerebral artery with absence of angular, posterior parietal and central sulcus arteries. (It is possible that these arose from a common trunk and were all involved by one large embolic fragment.) There is a gross occlusion of the pericallosal artery, the point of occlusion being rounded rather than tapered. Enough contrast passes this point to faintly outline the filling defect, representing an embolic fragment in the lumen.

A later film (B) shows filling of the central veins and contrast remaining in several arterial branches. This is especially prominent in the operculofrontal area, where arterial branches seen on the first film remain almost unchanged.

Stasis such as this is explained by occlusion of the tiny distal ramifications, leaving the visible portion of the vessel intact but plugging its run-off.

This case fills all the criteria for intracranial embolization except for disappearance of the occlusive process.

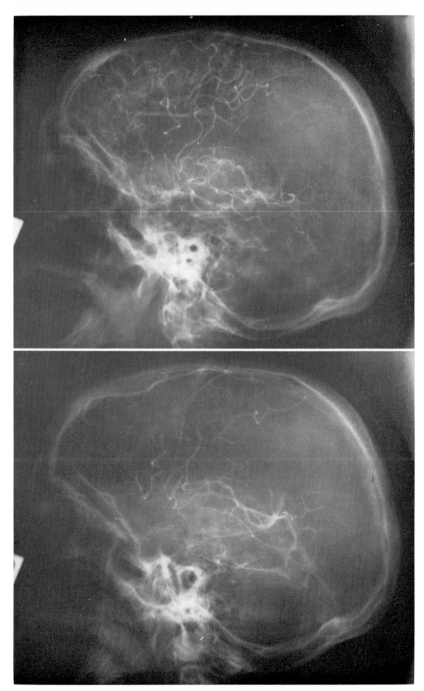

INTRACRANIAL EMBOLIZATION
32A (*Upper*), 32B (*Lower*).
See legend, page 109.

33. EMBOLIC OCCLUSIONS INVOLVING MIDDLE AND PERICALLOSAL ARTERIES

This patient is a pedagogic paradise of both normal and pathological anatomy. This 65-year-old male diabetic developed weakness in the left leg and later noted thickness of speech. An EEG showed slow activity anteriorly and posterior on the right.

The lateral view of the neck shows a filling defect in the carotid sinus with an irregularity on the upper portion of the defect that is characteristic of a small mural thrombus projecting into the lumen.

Intracranially, there is fairly obvious absence of the posterior parietal branch. Small vessels near the area of occlusion were excessively prominent on the original radiographs, but the occluded segment did not become opacified by retrograde collateral.

The central sulcus artery arises independently and is enfolded under the operculum, making the characteristic loop as it goes posteriorly around the lip to enter the depths of the fissure. The two branches are widely divergent, reaching to the anterior and posterior limits of the pre- and post-central gyri, a perfectly normal variant.

Turning to the pericallosal vessels, there is a good sized pericallosal artery that has a high course in its distal portion and sends a large branch to the posterior part of the paracentral lobule. However, there is only a tiny twig to the area just behind the coronal suture. Irrespective of where and how the blood supply of the paracentral lobule arises, one branch always enters from in front. With this in mind, the diagnosis of occlusion is obvious.

Note the small accessory branch to the corpus callosum that is often present when the pericallosal artery runs high in the interhemispheric fissure. The callosomarginal artery, or branches simulating it that run in the cingulate sulcus do not cross the marginal ramus but the pericallosal artery itself does even when running as high as the cingulate sulcus. The pericallosal artery in this case terminates with good sized branches in the precuneus and the last branch anterior to the precuneus outlines the marginal ramus. The relationship of this landmark to the central sulcus artery and the extension of the line separating posterior parietal and central sulcus areas is shown on the drawing.

The correlation between location of occlusions and neurological findings is better than many cases with embolic occlusions, probably because in the presence of emboli there are often more areas involved than are appreciated. This is also an example of the predominance of motor signs when multiple areas are involved. The leg weakness in this patient was the presenting difficulty, both to the patient and his physician, somewhat masking the symptoms arising from the second occlusion.

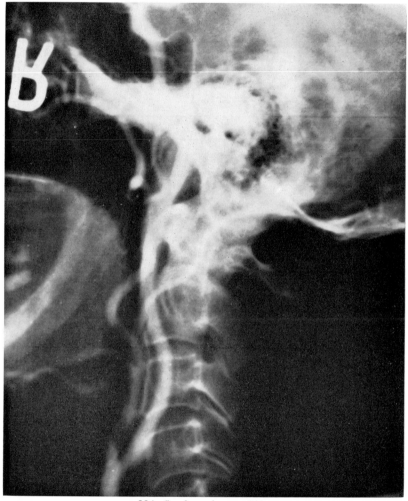

33A. See legend, page 111.

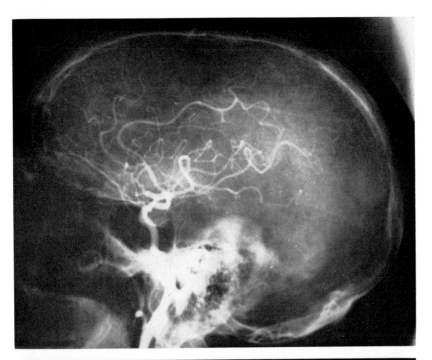

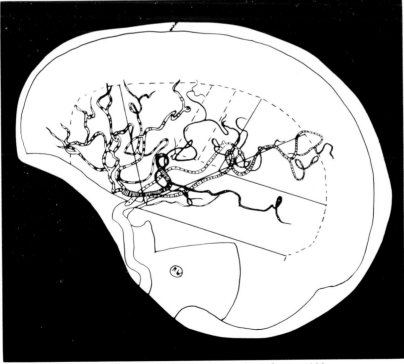

33B (*Upper*), 33C (*Lower*). See legend, page 111.

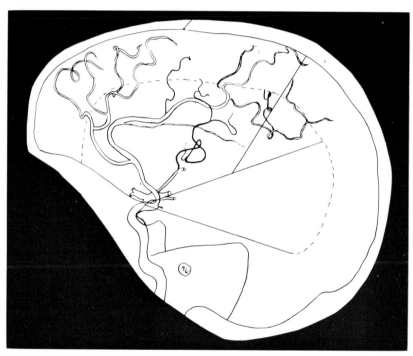

33D. Drawing of pericallosal arteries with the central sulcus artery of the middle cerebral included for reference. There are large branches to the posterior portion of the paracentral lobule but only a tiny twig in front diagnostic of an occlusion. See legend, page 111.

34. EMBOLIC OCCLUSION OF PORTION OF LATERAL BRANCH OF POSTERIOR CEREBRAL ARTERY DIAGNOSED BY VERTEBRAL ANGIOGRAPHY

Clinically, this patient was thought to have had a small stroke involving the temporal lobe and a carotid angiogram was planned. The examination, done by a house officer, resulted in an inadvertent but diagnostic vertebral study. There is an irregular stenosis in the vertebral artery just below the level of the foramen magnum, seen on both frontal and lateral projections (A,B) and the occluded stubs of branches from the temporal division of the posterior cerebral artery are seen on the frontal projection and outlined by arrows on the drawing. (C)

In all probability, the intracranial occlusions are due to emboli from the diseased segment of the vertebral artery. The vertebral artery has been found to be the source of posterior fossa emboli on postmortem material by several investigators, but the process is seldom documented angiographically.

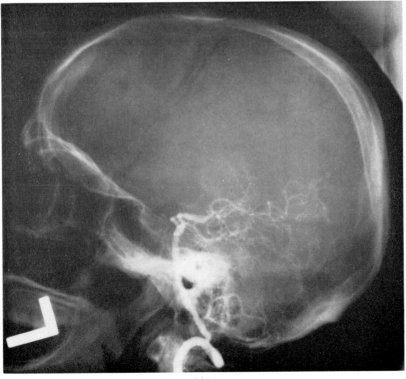

34A.

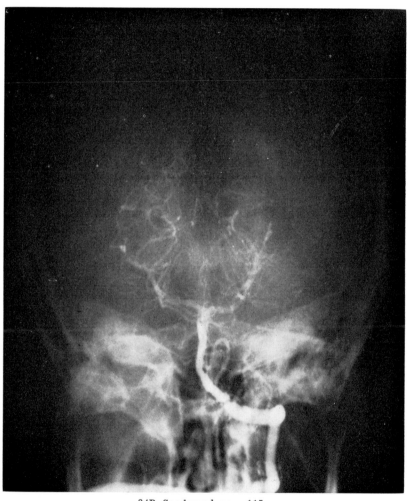

34B. See legend, page 115.

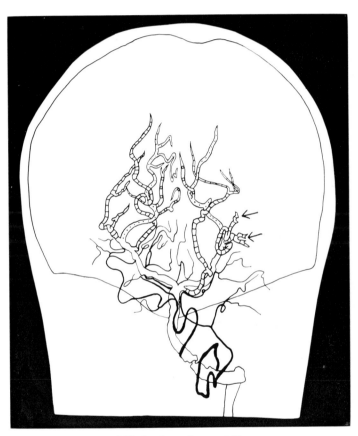

34C. See legend, page 115.

Generalized Embolization

Several, or occasionally all, previously listed criteria are present. There is usually a very characteristic picture with marked delay in circulation time but differing from the findings in extreme increased intracranial pressure in that the proximal arteries are normal or dilated.

35. GENERALIZED INTRACRANIAL EMBOLIZATION

This patient was a 55-year-old woman with an acute stroke and a rapidly progressing downhill course.

On a later film, there is a typical picture (A) with multiple occlusions, delayed circulation time and all evidence indicating intracranial emboli. On the enlargement of the earlier film, there is a filling defect in the internal carotid that projects into the lumen of the posterior cerebral largely occluding it. It is likely that the source of the emboli was a mural thrombus in the carotid siphon although it is impossible to be certain. No other sources of emboli were discovered and the carotid bifurcation appeared normal. (Reprinted by courtesy of *Amer. J. Roentgenol.*)

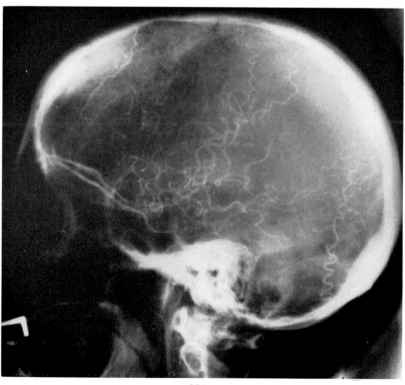

35A.

Microscopic Embolization

Emboli too small to occlude visible vessels are undetectable unless very numerous, in which case there is a delay in circulation time in the involved area. We have seen one extreme case in which the terminal arterioles were completely blocked by tumor cells, embolic from malignant melanoma. The circulation was so obstructed that injection into either carotid or vertebral artery refluxed down the other side and intravascular contrast was visible forty-five seconds after injection.

Most of the criteria need no explanation. Although emboli do occur in the presence of intracranial arterioclerosis, multiple arterio-sclerotic occlusions without visible evidence of arteriosclerosis in the remaining intracerebral vessels does not. The third criteria, the rounded end of the occluded vessel, is most helpful in recent or concomittant

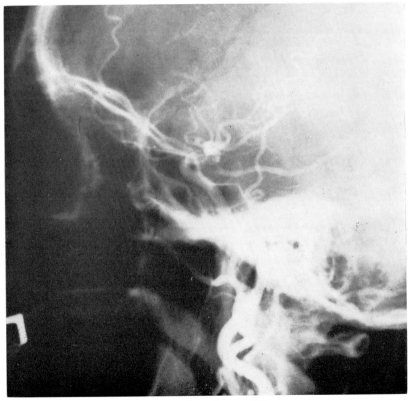

35B. See legend, page 118.

36. GENERALIZED INTRACRANIAL OCCLUSION WITH MICRO EMBOLI

Microemboli produce angiographic changes only if they are numerous enough to effect blood flow in the visible vessels. In this case, the distal arterial branches were so completely choked that the cerebral circulation was almost at a standstill and injection of contrast in one carotid caused reflux down the other. The proximal vessels are normal or dilated as opposed to the delayed circulation time with increased intracranial pressure. The emboli in this case were tumor cells of a malignant melanoma.

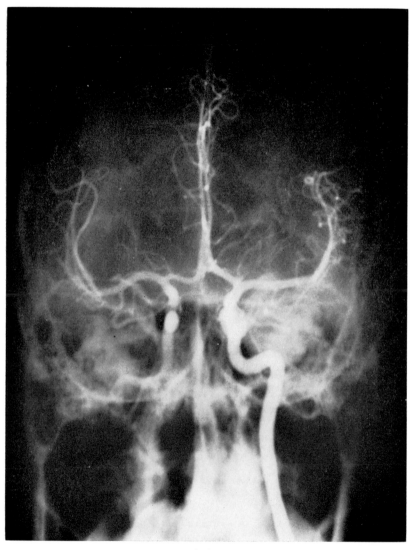

36A.

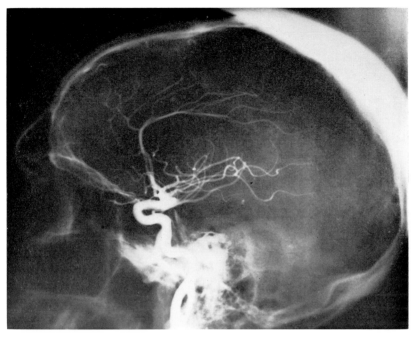

36B. See legend, page 120.

emboli since the point of occlusion is seldom obvious after the embolus stabilizes. The disappearance of an occlusion is quite diagnostic of an embolus if it occurs in a short time, but, as thrombotic occlusions may recanalize eventually and emboli of atheromatous debris cannot be expected to lyse, the time element and type of embolic material must be considered. A known source of emboli is very helpful and the carotid sinus must be carefully studied for minor irregularities that represent small mural thrombi.

Concealed Emboli

We introduced this term on the basis of the angiographic findings, but it has been well known to neuropathologists for some time and was described as "local embolism" by Fisher and colleagues and "forward embolism" by Loeb and Meyers. In this condition, a large mural thrombus embolizes and then, perhaps due to reflex spasm or diminished blood flow if a major intracranial trunk is occluded by the embolus, the thrombus extends to occlude the entire artery. Unless there is abundant intracranial collateral from the external

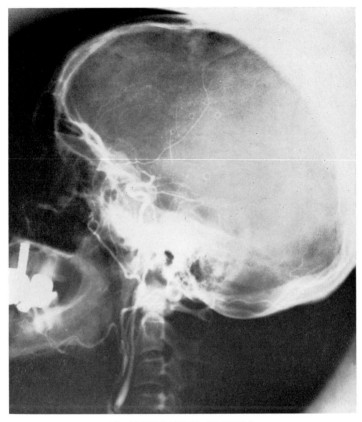

37. CONCEALED EMBOLI

The sudden diminution of flow in the carotid by embolization to a major intracranial artery may favor extension of a previously existing mural thrombus and lead to complete carotid occlusion. Since the carotid occlusion is abrupt, collateral from external to internal branches has not developed sufficiently to opacify the intracranial vessels and the intracranial occlusion is not detectable.

The case shown here is of interest in that there is enough contrast passing the thrombus to show some intracranial filling. The internal carotid is very small and there is faint opacification of the posterior cerebral, anterior choroid and pericallosal vessels, but the middle cerebral artery is completely occluded. A soft friable thrombus was removed from the carotid bifurcation at surgery. It is easy to see that with a little more time the carotid could be expected to close completely and the patient's stroke labelled another case of carotid thrombosis. The patient was only 41 years old and most of the cases of concealed emboli that we have encountered are in the younger age group. These patients in general have shown little evidence of generalized vascular disease and the process appears to be a local secondary effect of atherosclerosis that is especially tragic in view of its effect on an otherwise healthy and vigorous

$\longrightarrow$

carotid, which is not usually the case in sudden occlusions, or the contralateral carotid or a vertebral is studied, the intracranial occlusion is concealed by the extracranial one. This should be considered in patients with carotid occlusion in whom the clinical course is unusually acute and severe, particularly when occurring in the younger age group.

Small Intracerebral Hemorrhages

Although this work concerns occlusive rather than hemorrhagic processes the small intracerebral hemorrhages are mentioned as they may present with a clinical picture simulating embolic occlusions. The small hemorrhages arise from microaneurysms of the small arteries deep in the basal ganglia or white matter and are found in severe hypertensives. The small size of the vessel involved makes an angiographic diagnosis impossible unless the hematoma becomes large enough to cause displacement. This condition may be challenging to the clinician, as hypertensives may both bleed and embolize and the accepted treatment for one is highly undesirable for the other. (Recent reports by Mishkin and Leeds and Goldberg indicate that newer magnification techniques may reveal the lesions responsible for these small hemorrhages in some cases.)

---

individual. Both men and women have been encountered with this process, both before and after the introduction of "the pill" (oral contraceptives).

A small carotid distal to a major stenosis is a function of reduced blood flow and although congenitally small and atretic internal carotids do occur they are so rare that they should only be diagnosed after exclusion of all other possibilities. (Reprinted by courtesy of *Amer. J. Roentgenol., Rad. Ther. & Nucl. Med.*)

SECTION 15

INTRACRANIAL COLLATERAL, CONCEALED AND ASYMPTOMATIC OCCLUSIONS AND BORDER ZONE INFARCTS

COLLATERAL CIRCULATION to the brain may achieve the same goal, which is adequate perfusion of brain tissue, irrespective of the route employed. However, the angiographic appearance of collateral from extracranial arteries and intracranial source is entirely different, and unless this is thoroughly understood, may lead to erroneous interpretation of angiographic findings.

When collateral circulation from external to internal carotid in the presence of internal carotid occlusion—using the ophthalmic artery, the most common source, as an example—the collateral vessels function exactly as the internal carotid. The middle cerebral artery on the affected side becomes opacified but ordinarily the pericallosals do not as with only a minimal pressure gradient they will be filled from the other side. Good filling of both pericallosal groups in these circumstances indicates either an atretic anterior cerebral on the opposing side, a contralateral occlusive process with low pressure in the contralateral carotid, or occlusion of the middle cerebral itself. If the collateral from the external sources is not well developed, contrast in the main trunk of the middle cerebral will be diluted by blood entering from the opposite side or through the posterior communicating artery and it is impossible to assess the patency of the middle cerebral branches. If the collateral is well developed, it balances the pressure from the remainder of the circle

38. CONCEALED OCCLUSIONS

In the presence of a chronic stenosing process of the internal carotid, collateral circulation may develop effectively enough to prevent symptoms. This collateral may be seen going from external to internal branches, most commonly through the ophthalmic artery. The pericallosal vessels on the involved side are usually supplied by the opposing carotid, and the area supplied by this artery may be expected to extend toward the low pressure area so that the blood flow in the middle cerebral branches is considerably reduced, although the brain is still perfused sufficiently to maintain normal metabolism. However, the reduced blood flow by itself, in the presence of the same degenerative processes that caused the carotid occlusion, predisposes to thrombosis. When the patient, who has been existing on his collateral circulation for some time, develops an intracranial occlusion and has angiography the carotid thrombosis is so obvious that the deficiency in the indirectly opacified intracranial branches is overlooked.

The first patient was a 61-year-old man who suddenly developed aphasia and hemiparesis. The hemiparesis improved but the aphasia persisted. The left carotid angiogram shows complete carotid occlusions (A) and fairly prompt opacification of the carotid siphon by way of a large ophthalmic artery and most of the middle cerebral artery branches (B).

Details are better seen on the drawing (C) where there is a prominent orbito-frontal branch. The central sulcus artery and all branches behind it are intact but there is complete absence of the operculofrontal artery.

The second patient was a 70-year-old man who had not felt entirely well for a month and who had vague complaints for a week prior to a typical stroke resulting in hemiparesis. By the time he was examined, there was no aphasia and paralysis was confined to the arm.

The carotid abnormalities are a little more unusual. The internal carotid shows a stenosis and filling defect in the sinus (D) but contrast passes upward to stop abruptly at the beginning of a right angle bend so that the vessel seen on a later film (E) resembles a stand pipe. On this same film, there is opacification of the carotid siphon through a large ophthalmic artery. The carotid occlusion in this individual is probably at the site of a kink or arteriosclerotic plaque in a congenital loop in the artery and it is quite possible that this represents lodgment of an embolus from a mural thrombus at the bifurcation. The efficiency of the collateral through the ophthalmic, however, indicates that a severe stenosis has been present for a long period of time.

On a later film (F), there is good filling of the middle cerebral artery branches with the exception of the central sulcus artery. This is seen arising more proximally than usual and coming to an abrupt end. This is shown in solid black on the drawing (G).

It is quite likely that the occlusion in the latter case represented a fragment that embolized intracranially before the carotid was completely occluded. In the first case, however, the process was almost certainly a primary thrombosis. Both cases show excellent correlation between neurological findings and the areas involved by the occlusions.

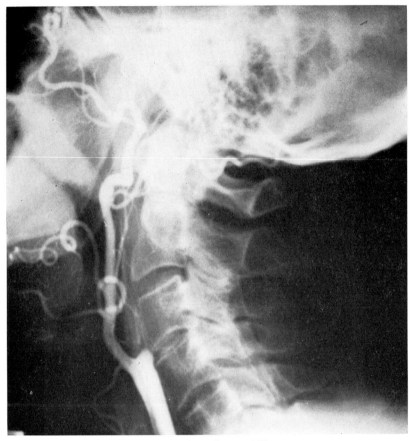

38A. See legend, page 125.

of Willis and the branches are accurately and completely opacified, exactly as though the internal carotid were patent, the only difference being a slight delay in filling. It is probable that the total area irrigated is reduced circumferentially provided the other carotid and basilar circulations are normal, but any reduction occurs in the area of the tiny distal ramifications and is not apparent on films. This means, very simply, that with good collateral from the external carotid, all branches of the middle cerebral artery will be visible if patent and, if not visible, are occluded.

Collateral circulation developing after intracranial occlusions or severe stenosis of intracranial arteries is an entirely different matter. Taveras and Wood discuss this thoroughly in their text. This occurs

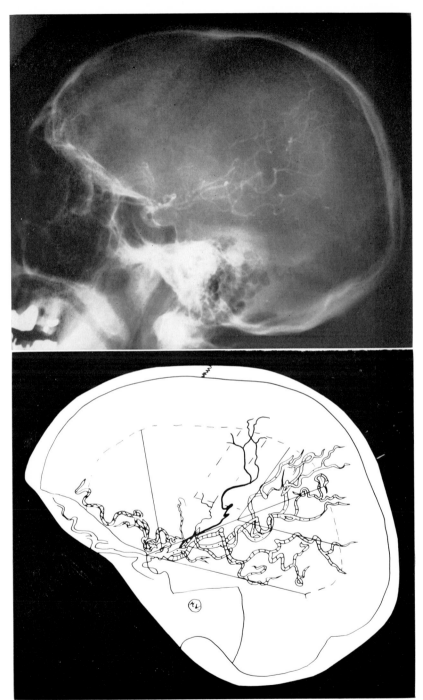

38B (*Upper*), 38C (*Lower*). See legend, page 125.

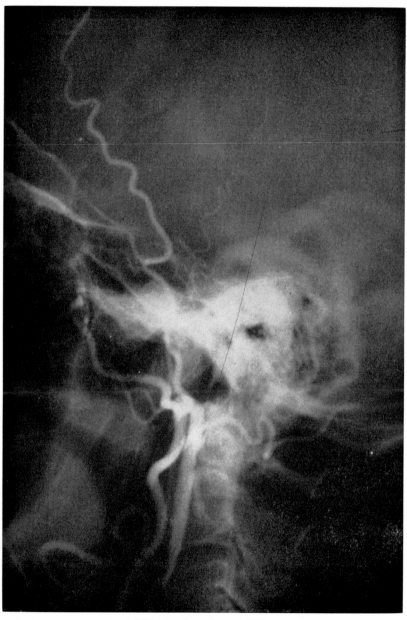

38D. See legend, page 125.

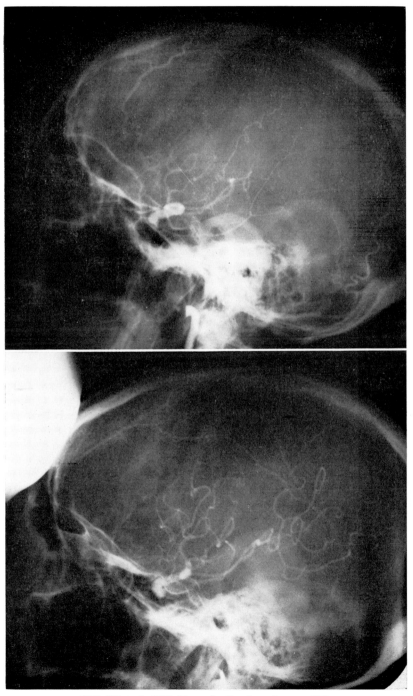

38E (*Upper*), 38F (*Lower*). See legend, page 125.

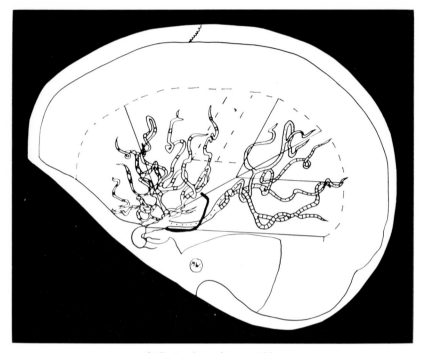

38G. See legend, page 125.

through the small distal anastomotic communications and flows in retrograde manner from a low pressure area to a normally higher pressured one, running up hill so to speak. The distance that this collateral travels through visible arteries depends entirely on the pressure at the two ends and due to the multiplicity of the connections cannot be expected to be identical in all parts of the involved areas. Consequently, retrograde collateral filling is seldom complete and symmetrical and the degree of filling or nonfilling of individual branches cannot be used to either diagnose or exclude additional occlusions distal to the primary process. When complete occlusion of a major intracranial artery occurs, the extent of visible collateral depends on the contrast in the adjacent vessels and will appear more extensive if the posterior cerebral is opacified than if it is not. This collateral is seen as a positive density in the vessels that are filled. In the presence of a severe stenosis instead of an occlusion, some contrast containing blood passes the stenosis with reduced pressure and flows

39. ASYMPTOMATIC INTRACRANIAL STENOSIS: INCOMPLETE FILLING DUE TO RETROGRADE COLLATERAL

This 49-year-old patient was examined because of a questionable retro-orbital mass and had no neurological abnormalities whatsoever.

On the frontal projection, there is a marked stenosis of the main trunk of the middle cerebral artery. On both frontal and lateral projections, there is only filling of the proximal portions of some of the middle cerebral branches and contrast seemed to stand still in the intracranial vessels, later opacifying the deep veins in fairly normal manner. The lack of filling of the branches is due to retrograde blood flow from pericallosal and posterior cerebral arteries.

The patient's exopthalmos eventually was decided to be due to an unusual form of thyroid over-activity.

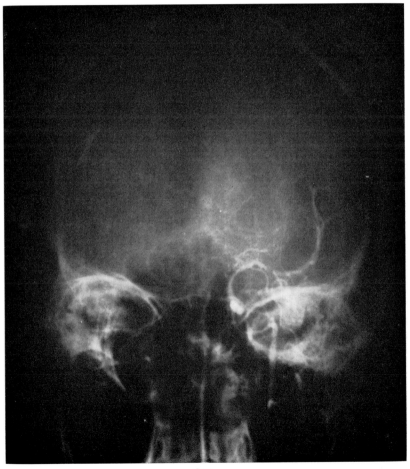

39A.

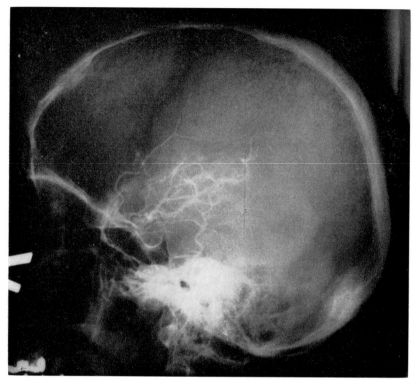

39B. See legend, page 131.

out into the branches until its pressure is equalized by the retrograde collateral flow. This is seen as a negative density or lack of filling of the distal branches and on a single film may superficially resemble generalized embolization and multiple occlusions. It is important that these two conditions are not confused as the prognosis and clinical course differ in the extreme.

This prepares the way to the diagnosis of concealed intracranial occlusions that are not necessarily embolic. Intracranial occlusions occur and can be diagnosed by angiography in cases of chronic occlusion of the internal carotid in which the involved hemisphere is supplied by an efficient collateral from the external carotid branches. It is doubtful if such occlusions are embolic since likely sources of emboli are excluded and would tend to be filtered out by circuitous route and small size of the collateral anastomoses, and are more likely primary thromboses on the basis of pre-existing arteriosclerosis. Anything temporarily lowering the intracranial blood flow would, as in Denny-Brown's concept, predispose to such a thrombosis. The important thing in these cases is to recognize the intracranial occlusion which can be done by applying anatomical principles as in any other case and not to consider the long standing carotid occlusion as the agent responsible for the recent stroke. Having made this mistake several times in the past, we are especially sensitized to it.

The matter of asymptomatic occlusions is intimately related to intracranial collateral. We have had no experience with what can honestly be called an asymptomatic intracranial occlusion, the nearest to it is the severe middle cerebral artery stenosis in Figure 39 in which angiography was done for a question of retro-orbital tumor and no neurological deficit was present. It has been long recognized that extracranial occlusions may be multiple and asymptomatic and intracranial occlusions are not infrequently incidental findings in association with other intracranial processes or found on postoperative examinations. In the latter cases, the manifestations are masked by the primary disease process and one cannot say whether or not they would have been asymptomatic in themselves. Accidental postoperative occlusions may have no residua, but again it is impossible to be sure that they would have been asymptomatic under other conditions. The recovery potential is sometimes amazing and may occur spontaneously in the postoperative period while the patient is obtunded from surgery and any additional neurological deficit is not recognizable. We have been impressed by the minimal neurological changes in some cases of what appear to be gross disease, such as the patient in Figure 39, as opposed to the severe hemiparesis in patients with occlusion of only the central sulcus artery in whom the angiogram can be readily passed as normal. The differences are due to the acuteness of the process and the rapidity with which intracranial collateral enlarges, and are not so amazing if one remembers that the blood in vessels big enough to be seen angiographically is actually playing no part in brain metabolism. If the tiny vessels that supply the individual cells are adequately perfused, which is possible in the presence of gradual occlusions, the status of the larger arteries is immaterial. The reason more evidence of asymptomatic intracranial occlusions is not available

is probably due to the fact that intracranial, as opposed to extracranial occlusions, seldom develop as slowly progressive stenoses.

Border zone infarcts, described as water shed infarcts by Fisher,
are mentioned only because of their relationship with intracranial
collateral as they cannot be diagnosed angiographically. The three
major intracerebral trunks supply definite areas and at the borders
of these areas the distal vascular ramifications overlap and intermingle.
Blood flows peripherally in these small vessels until it is hydraulically
balanced by flow in the opposite direction from adjoining vessels.
The border zone between the major arterial complexes is not rigidly
fixed and if the effective pressure in one component is slightly lowered
there is an increase flow toward the lower pressure area until the
system is again in balance. If, however, there is a drop in effective
forward pressure in more than one or in all the intracerebral trunks,
the flow in the distal branches is limited by its internal resistance
rather than equalized hydraulic forces and the total area supplied by
the involved trunks shrinks about the periphery leaving zones between
them in which the blood in the distal branches does not flow in either
direction. If the stasis is prolonged, occlusive platelet aggregates and
infarctions develop. This is commonly seen in association with extracranial stenoses or occlusions or generalized intracerebral arteriosclerosis but may be precipitated or even occur in the presence of
normal vessels by severe and prolonged hypotension such as in surgical
shock.

---

40. ASYMPTOMATIC (?) OCCLUSION, POSTOPERATIVE

A young man with pronounced vascular displacement from a large astro-
cytoma. The angular branch bifurcates with a prominent inferior branch.
Even in the presence of this displacement, the central sulcus artery and, as
a result, the location of the motor strip can be identified. The central sulcus
artery is the last branch of the ascending frontal complex, arising just in front
of the divergence of the three posterior major trunks.

After surgery, the prominent inferior branch of the angular artery has
disappeared. The patient had persistence of hemianopsia, but this would be
expected in view of the extent of surgery necessary to remove the tumor.
Occlusions of a "branch of a branch" such as this cannot be ordinarily diagnosed by angiography and it is questionable whether this occlusion would have
given significant symptoms if it had occurred as a primary event in the presence
of otherwise healthy vessels. Such minor occlusions may be significant in
the presence of generalized arteriosclerosis or a generalized reduction in cerebral
blood flow from any other cause.

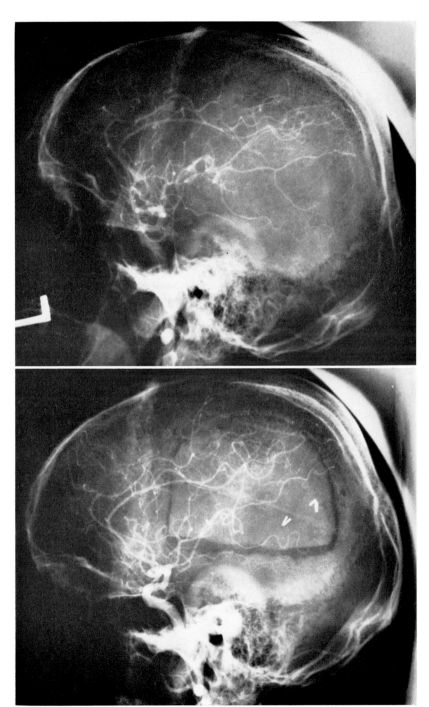

40A (*Upper*), 40B (*Lower*). See legend, page 134.

The distal ramifications of the middle cerebral and pericallosal arteries overlap at the level of the superior frontal gyrus and the infarcts are commonly found along this plane. The motor strip at this level controls trunk and hip movements and, clinically, the patients may have difficulty in walking since they are unable to stabilize the trunk, although their leg muscles are perfectly normal.

The presence of border zone infarcts is more a matter for clinical than angiographic diagnosis as the angiogram can do no more than demonstrate the underlying vascular processes leading to their occurrence—either extracranial stenoses or occlusions and/or generalized intracranial arteriosclerosis. This is a valuable concept but there is the possibility of improper usage since it is much easier to write off an angiogram without gross abnormalities as negative and attribute the symptoms to a border zone infarct rather than to expend the effort necessary to find an occlusion of a visible branch.

SECTION 16

LIMITATIONS OF ANGIOGRAPHY

Even under the best of conditions, not all intracranial occlusions can be diagnosed angiographically. What can and should be done is to improve the percentage. In most series of angiograms on stroke patients, the number with "normal" examinations is about 50%. In our recent experience, the number of stroke patients with normal angiograms is about 10% and by taking only those cases in whom a discharge diagnosis of cerebral thrombosis or embolism was recorded, Waddington found only 10 normal studies in 252 patients (4%). The difference between the 10% and the 4% is largely due to the exclusion of patients in the latter group in whom a diagnosis of occlusive cerebrovascular disease was suspected but never proved. Some patients in this category turn up later with definite cerebrovascular disease and in others there is a wide range of conditions from neurasthenia to neoplasia.

The factors responsible for a lack of diagnostic findings can be summarized as follows:
1. Incomplete or technically unsatisfactory examination. This is discussed under technique and is self-explanatory.
2. Occlusions of cortical vessels too small to be seen angiographically.
   A. *Transient ischemic attacks*: If these episodes are caused by tiny platelet emboli, the occlusions involve vessels too small to be seen. If the episodes are due to the hemodynamic crises of Denny-Brown, the extracranial stenoses or occlusions are obvious. A stenosis can only be considered significant if it

[137]

involves at least 50% of the diameter of an extracranial
vessel and it is unlikely that a stenosis no greater than this
would cause symptoms unless several vessels were similarly
involved. Some cases show minor irregularities in the carotid
sinus that represent the source of tiny intracranial emboli
but, although this can be suspected, it is hard to prove when
no evidence of intracranial occlusion exists.

B. *Infarctions with permanent changes*: This group includes
the border zone infarcts and, while not recognizable by themselves, the factors responsible for their production—severe
stenosing arteriosclerosis of the extra- or intracranial vessels
and/or the history of an episode of marked hypotension—are
not likely to be overlooked.

3. Occlusion of the penetrating arteries causing deep infarcts. In
the past, this was thought to be the most common cause of stroke.
Although our experience suggests that this occurs in no more
and probably much less than 10% of stroke patients, it does
occur as an isolated event and to date is impossible to diagnose
angiographically. Krayenbuhl and Yarsagil noted that the clinical
course in patients with middle cerebral artery occlusion was much
more severe when the occlusion involved the lenticulostriate arteries
than when they were spared.

4. Lysis of an embolus prior to angiography. It is doubtful if this is
a factor if angiography is performed as soon as the patient's condition stabilizes since an embolus big enough to cause an infarct
would not be expected to disappear within a week or two, but it
is a real possibility if angiography is delayed a month or more.

5. Undetected occlusions of cortical branches. This is undoubtedly
the primary cause of the generally unsatisfactory numbers of
definitive diagnoses in stroke patients. Not all occlusions of reason-
ably good sized cortical branches can be recognized, but the numbers missed can be greatly diminished by careful study and a detailed knowledge of vascular anatomy.

We are never entirely happy with a diagnosis of intracranial arteriosclerosis in patients with an acute stroke but have had to accept it in
about 10% of cases (29 of 252 patients in Waddington's series).
There is no question but that infarcts occur with generalized intra-

cranial arteriosclerosis without occlusion of angiographically visible vessels, the problem being that this is not a definitive radiographic diagnosis as the arteriosclerosis may exist and be found as an incidental in patients without symptoms of occlusive cerebrovascular disease. In the absence of a more specific finding, there is always the possibility that the primary disease process, such as occlusions of visible branches, a small intracerebral hematoma or an early glioma, has been missed. Since some degree of degenerative change in the intracranial vessels is common in the older age groups, intracranial arteriosclerosis can be accepted as a cause for symptoms only when it is definite and generalized. The use of a hand lens is helpful in differentiating insignificant tortuosity and possible flattening of a vessel in one plane from the multiple stenoses and luminal irregularities of generalized intracranial arteriosclerosis.

The specific type of arteriosclerosis involving the subcortical vessels, resulting in Binzwanger's syndrome, is an entity by itself and has little in common with the occlusive processes discussed here.

TECHNIQUE

A WORD CONCERNING technique is in order since a diagnosis based on anatomical detail is impossible if radiographic detail is wanting. There are many variations in the techniques of cerebral angiography but the goal of all should be the maximum diagnostic information with the least possible discomfort and danger to the patient and the methods used may vary from one institution to another depending on individual skill and experience. It is doubtful if any one method is sufficiently superior to any other to warrant changing a routine that works well and is thoroughly familiar. In our experience direct carotid puncture gives the most information with the least morbidity although if generalized cerebrovascular disease is suspected it is usually preceded by mapping the great vessels with a catheter injection. We use the basic technique acquired from Lindgren in Stockholm in which a sharp needle is used and the vessel punctured rather than threaded and a constant slow injection of saline without heparin carried on to prevent clotting. We have found it advantageous to connect a three-way stopcock to the adapter between needle and syringe and obtain the saline from a suspended intravenous bottle. This insures sterility, reduces the number of personnel required, and allows an uninterrupted saline injection that has been effective in preventing clotting in the needle with subsequent embolization. Carotid studies are done with local anesthesia in all patients able to cooperate but in others, especially stroke victims, the possible hazard of general anesthesia seems less than the hazard of badly traumatizing an artery which is likely to happen in a restless, squirming patient. At times, the arterial outlines on angiograms are vague and ill defined without obvious reason and although this is more common in young patients without increased intracranial pressure on whom the examination is done under general anesthesia, it is occasionally found in patients with intracranial pathology, making an anatomical diagnosis difficult. This apparently is due to intravascular streaming of contrast associated with a rapid circulation and the improvement in film quality after hyperventilation, as suggested by Du Boulay, is dramatic whether the patient is anesthetized or not and is heartily recommended. Since intracranial conditions in which hyperventilation may be hazardous are hardly compatible with a generalized excessively rapid cerebral circulation time, the presence of poor quality films for this reason is in itself evidence that hyperventilation can be safely and advantageously used.

Subintimal or pervascular injections are much more hazardous to the patient with cerebrovascular disease than to those with other conditions and by artificially altering hemodynamics conceal valuable information so that angiography in stroke patients is preferably done by the experienced angiographer. It is wise to avoid the carotid sinus in puncturing the artery due to the danger of embolization rather than any possible carotid sinus reflex, and the puncture should be made low enough to show the bifurcation. In patients with short necks, or when using some film changes, an additional "long neck" lateral view by placing a film down over the shoulder is necessary to show the area. The carotid bifurcation is so often the source of intracranial emboli and technical errors in injection so prone to disturb existing flow patterns that the angiogram in the stroke patient cannot be considered complete unless it shows both the carotid bifurcation and the point of the needle. The use of a preliminary film with injection of a small amount of contrast is useful in checking the position of the needle and is especially recommended when angiography is performed by physicians in their training period.

Practically all apparatus for serial films, whether cassette, roll or cut film changers, have the potential of producing satisfactory films although hand-pulled cassettes consistently give detail that is seldom matched by any other method. Elaborate and expensive apparatus

41. SUBINTIMAL INJECTION OF CONTRAST SIMULATING INTERNAL
CAROTID OCCLUSION

This patient was quite ill, confused and restless, with a large malignant glioma. The frontal projection shows displacement by the tumor but a perfectly normal internal carotid. On lateral view, there is the characteristic appearance of subintimal injection. The very dense column of contrast with a rounded upper end represents the avulsed segment of intima with contrast under it. A minimal amount of contrast passes into the external carotid, while the internal is seen to come to a pointed end, simulating carotid thrombosis.

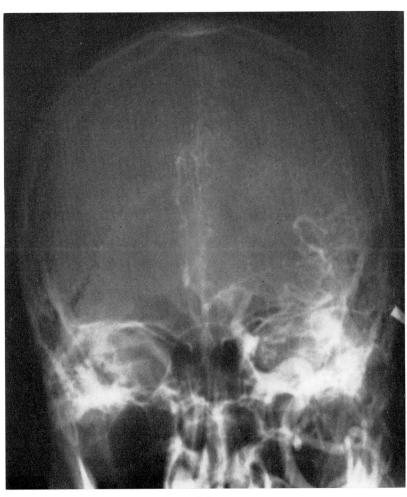

41A.

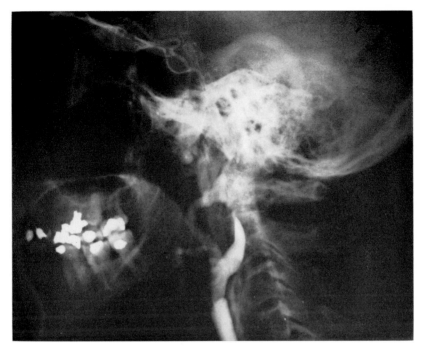

41B. See legend, page 142.

is not required but what is necessary, and sometimes harder to come by, is meticulous attention to all technical details so that the apparatus produces films at its optimum capability.

Vertebral angiography is mentioned only for completeness. An indirect approach by a catheter, subclavian or brachial injection, is desirable when examining patients with occlusive vascular disease of the vertebrobasilar system in order to locate or exclude gross lesions, as they often occur at the origin of the vertebrals and direct injection may be hazardous in the presence of basilar thrombosis. We find that direct vertebral injections give better intracranial detail and this is routine in suspected bleeds or tumors. General anesthesia is routine in direct vertebral angiography since the procedure is more likely to be painful and any movement by the patient more likely to dislodge the needle than in a carotid study.

SECTION 18

EXAMPLES OF OCCLUSIONS

The following section is similar to that portraying normal anatomy and represents examples of occlusions. These are shown in order of their relative frequency, the largest number are those involving the middle cerebral artery starting with the most anterior branches and progressing posteriorly. The anterior cerebral, pericallosal and posterior cerebral occlusions follow in this order. Various types of occlusive processes are included for the purpose of illustrating points that are discussed in the text. Not all possible types of occlusions are included, for example, sickle cell anemia. This disorder in northern New England is but little more common than the cerebral complications of malaria. In this series, some of the occlusions are quite obvious but others are not. When the vessels are properly identified and sorted out, as shown in the drawings, they are readily seen. The drawings serve as illustrations; the physician making the diagnosis must use his knowledge of anatomy to identify the various branches directly from the film.

42. OCCLUSION OF ORBITOFRONTAL ARTERY

Occlusion of the orbitofrontal artery as an isolated event is rare and this is the only example that we have encountered. The patient was a 62-year-old man who was examined because of a sudden and pronounced personality change, that can be briefly described as "frontal lobish."

The angiogram (A) shows prominent external vessels and a small pericallosal artery. The meningeal vessels outlining the middle fossa are unusually prominent and tend to conceal the absence of orbitofrontal branches. When the vessels are sorted out and the external branches omitted on the drawing (B), the absence of orbitofrontal branches is obvious. (Reprinted by courtesy of *Brain*.)

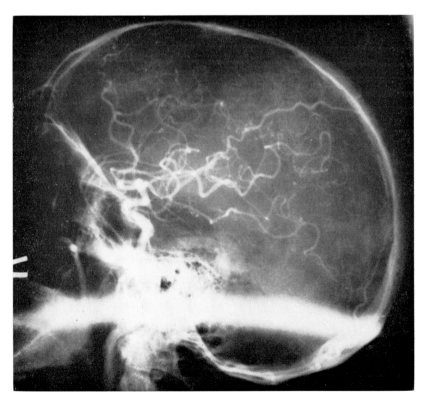

42A.

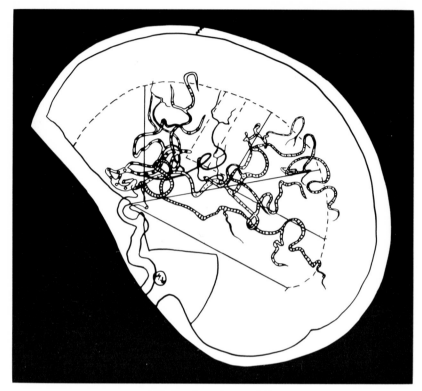

42B. See legend, page 145.

43. OCCLUSION OF ANTERIOR HALF OF OPERCULOFRONTAL BRANCH

This man had a stroke at age 70 with aphasia and right hemiparesis. The hemiparesis disappeared and the aphasia improved to a point that it was barely perceptible. Angiography was not performed until three years later when he was admitted following a seizure and was found to have had a subarachnoid hemorrhage.

On the left (angiogram and drawing), the orbitofrontal branches are intact but there is a sizable void between them and one good sized operculofrontal branch that bifurcates. Since any portion of the ascending frontal complex or individual branches of the three components may have separate origins, the occlusion of only part of the operculofrontal branches should not be surprising.

The pericallosal vessels are of interest. On the side of occlusion, there is a huge pericallosal artery with large branches that are doubly numerous posteriorly since this one artery supplies the precuneus on both sides. On the right side, the pericallosal is small and terminates in the paracentral lobule, the last branch running upward outlines the marginal ramus. The pericallosal itself supplies the posterior portion of the paracentral lobule and at the level of the coronal suture there is a prominent branch that supplies the anterior portion. The filling of both posterior cerebrals from the carotids suggests but is not diagnostic of a lowered pressure in the vertebrobasilar system. This patient's subsequent course indicated that this was not abnormal.

No bleeding point was found at angiography and clinically the patient did well.

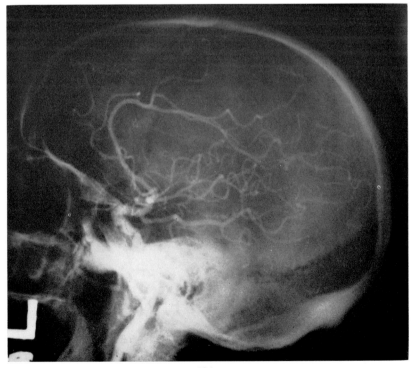

43A.

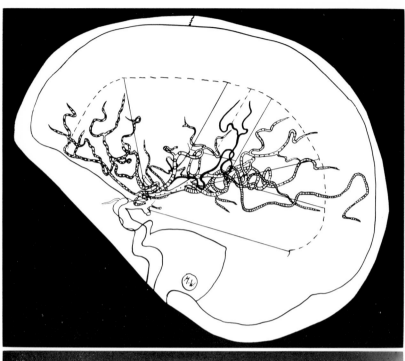

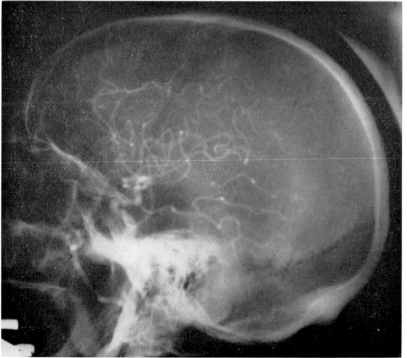

43B (*Upper*), 43C (*Lower*). See legend, page 147.

44. EDEMA ASSOCIATED WITH SMALL ARTERY OCCLUSION
OCCLUSION OF CENTRAL SULCUS ARTERY

There is often minimal distortion of vessels in the area adjacent to an infarct but occasionally, for no obvious reason, the displacement may be pronounced. This lady was examined a week after a stroke with resultant hemiparesis, most marked in the arm. The pericallosal vessels are normal but there is a large area devoid of vessels in the posterior opercula region. Identifying the vessels in a counter-clockwise direction, there is a large posterior temporal artery, a prominent angular that divides into two distal branches and a big posterior parietal artery. There is nothing in front of the posterior parietal artery until one meets two partially superimposed and abnormally straight operculofrontal branches that bifurcate distally. On the original radiographs, there are fine vessels surrounding this avascular area and the lenticulostriate vessels are unusually prominent. The vascular displacement is more obvious on the drawing and the operculofrontal artery appears to be intact.

The only definite occlusion is that of the central sulcus artery and apparently the vascular displacement is due only to unusually pronounced edema. In this particular case, the displacement serves to accentuate the absence of vessels but such displacements may be confusing and simulate tumor.

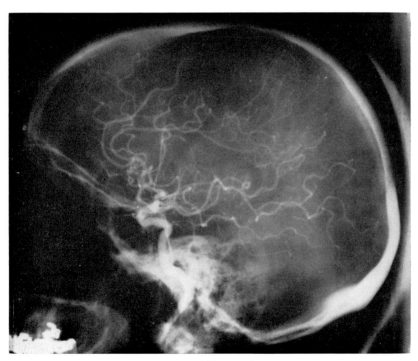

44A

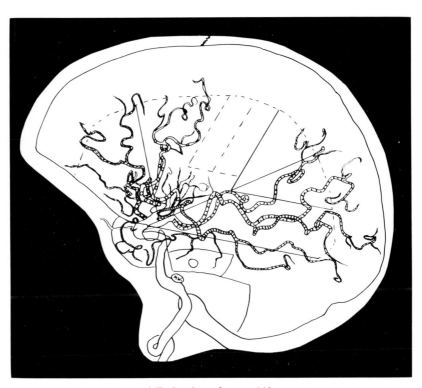

44B. See legend, page 149.

45. ARTERIAL STASIS DUE TO PRESSURE FROM SUBDURAL HEMATOMA

This young woman developed a marked hemiparesis after head injury. On the frontal projection, there is a small subdural hematoma following the convexity of the brain. The pericallosal arteries have largely emptied but most of the middle cerebral branches are still opacified.

On the lateral film, there is the same differential in circulation time, the pericallosal arteries are completely filled while the distal middle cerebral arteries are not. Of particular interest is the central sulcus artery. This arises from the operculofrontal group and makes the characteristic loop around the posterior lip of the operculum as it enters the depths of the fissure, but is only filled for a centimeter or so.

On a later film, residual contrast is seen in the distal ramifications of the posterior parietal, angular and posterior temporal arteries while the central sulcus artery remains well opacified at its origin and is still only filled for an inch or so. The visible dye column does not reach the bifurcation into anterior and posterior branches that always occur when only one central sulcus artery is present.

It is impossible to be sure that there was not a pre-existing stenosis or concurrent embolus to the central sulcus artery, but there was no history to suggest it. It is assumed that this stasis is only the result of pressure. At any rate, the unusually severe hemiparesis is without question related to the marked delayed circulation in this particular branch.

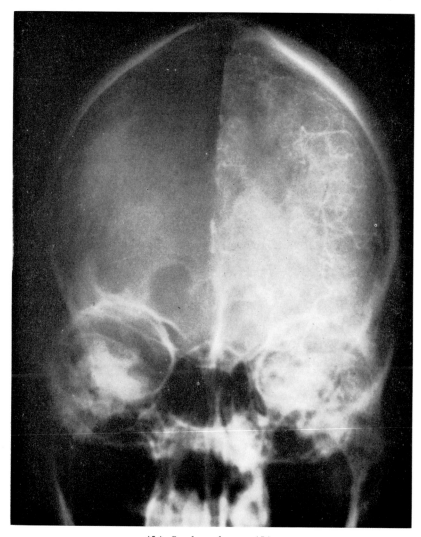

45A. See legend, page 151.

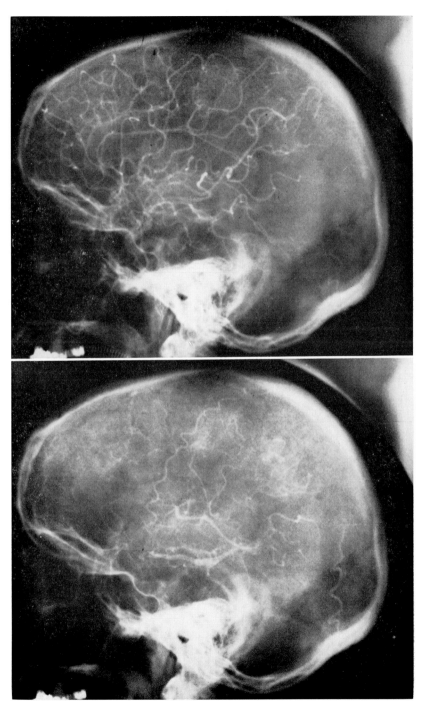

45B (*Upper*), 45B (*Lower*). See legend, page 151.

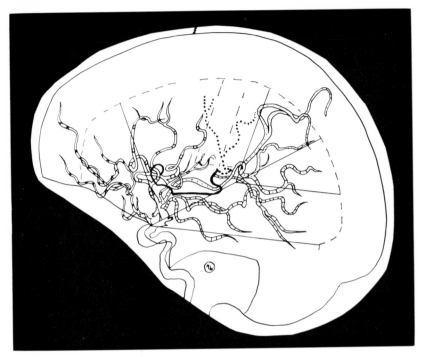

45C. See legend, page 151.

46. OCCLUSION OF POSTERIOR PARIETAL ARTERY DUE TO ARTERITIS

This 19-year-old girl had a sudden onset of left hemiparesis and was found to have right mid- and posterior EEG abnormalities. The clinical diagnosis was either vascular occlusion or an AV malformation.

There is good filling of pericallosal, middle and posterior cerebral arteries. On the frontal projection, there is a pronounced stenosis of the main trunk of the middle cerebral. On lateral views, more obvious on the drawing, in which only the middle cerebral artery branches are shown, there is complete absence of the posterior parietal branch. On the enlargement, the point of obstruction of the posterior parietal branch is visible and there is a long segment of severe stenosis of the central sulcus artery near its origin, there being only one central sulcus artery in this case. In the enlargement, note the beaded appearance of the branch supplying the posterior portion of the paracentral lobule (*arrows*). This portion of the pericallosal artery is included in the drawing.

The diagnosis of arteritis can be made on the basis of the beaded appearance of the artery alone. The elongated areas of stenosis are characteristic but less specific. In this case, the beaded appearance in one location, the elongated and multiple stenoses and the occlusion leave no doubt as to the diagnosis of arteritis. In the young female, such an arteritis is frequently a manifestation of lupus erythematosus.

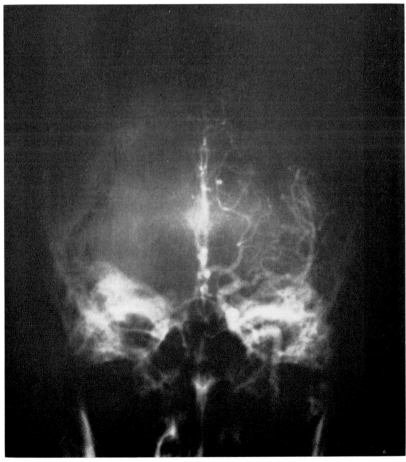

46A

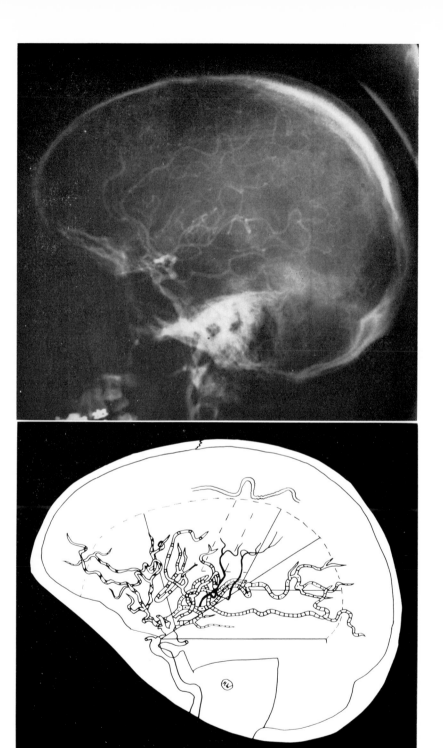

46B (*Upper*), 46C (*Lower*). See legend, page 155.

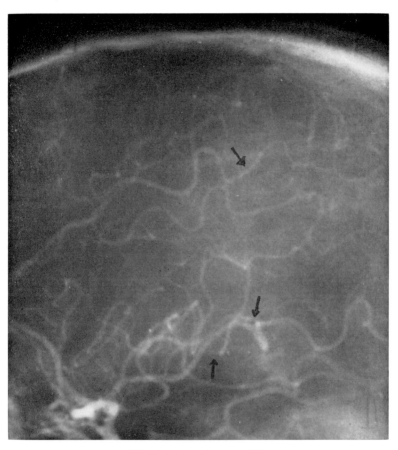

46D. See legend, page 155.

47. CORRELATION OF BRAIN SCAN AND ANGIOGRAM
OCCLUSION OF POSTERIOR PARIETAL ARTERY

A patient with clinical evidence of a parietal lobe lesion with absence of
the posterior parietal branch of the middle cerebral. The absence of this
branch is somewhat concealed by the distal pericallosal artery branches that
are especially numerous as both pericallosal arteries are filled from this side.
Films are shown with early and later arterial filling; the drawing emphasizes
the absence of the posterior parietal branch and the brain scan is shown with
the template superimposed, the area of uptake corresponding to the area supplied
by the posterior parietal artery. (Reprinted by courtesy of the *Amer. J. Med.*)

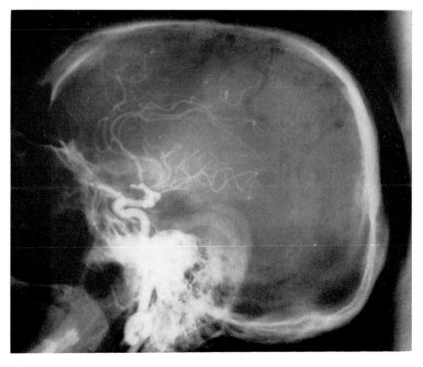

47A.

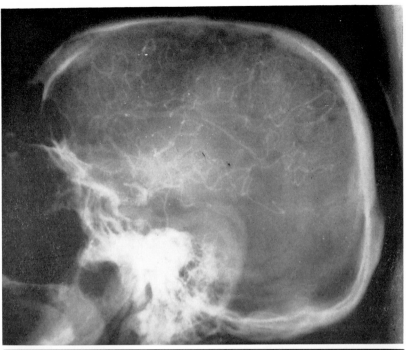

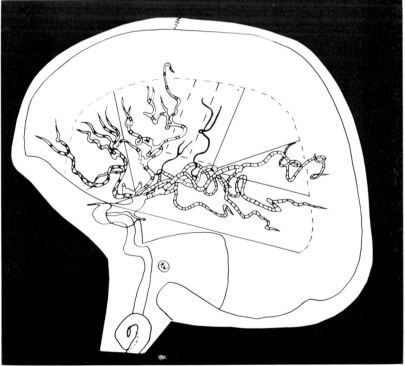

47B *(Upper)*, 47C *(Lower)*. See legend, page 158.

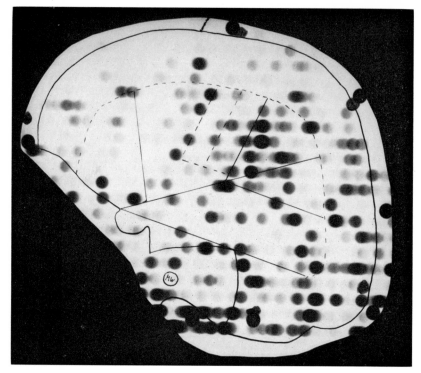

47D. See legend, page 158.

48. OCCLUSION OF ANGULAR ARTERY

This patient presented with symptoms more suggestive of a parietal lobe tumor than stroke, but angiography reveals complete absence of the angular artery. The posterior temporal artery is large and leaves the Sylvian fissure early as is found in about 15% of examinations. The central sulcus artery is unusual but not abnormal. It arises from the operculofrontal branch and runs posteriorly well above the level of the operculum and enters the Rolandic fissure fully an inch above its usual point of entry.

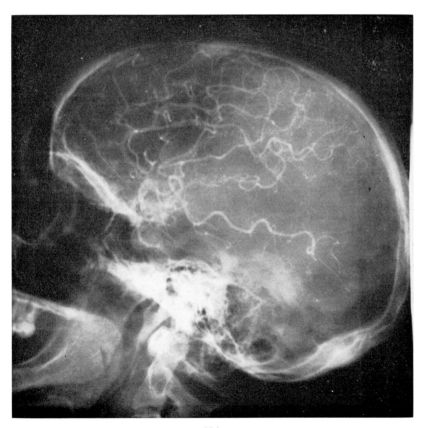

48A

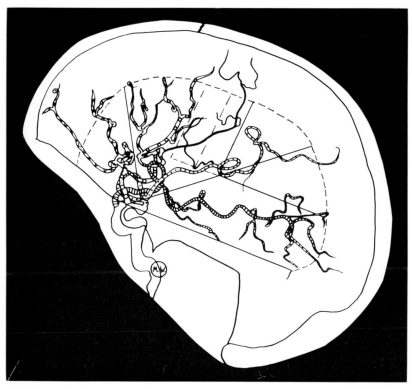

48B. See legend, page 161.

49. OCCLUSION OF POSTERIOR TEMPORAL ARTERY

This case was supplied by Doctor Waddington from St. Lukes Hospital in Utica, New York. The patient was a 42-year-old diabetic who developed anomia and transient parasthesias of the right arm. No visual field defect could be demonstrated. Bilateral angiograms were done and on the left side (A) there is complete absence of any significant branches to the posterior temporal area. The angular and posterior parietal arteries are large and prominent and better seen on the drawing (B). The central sulcus artery shows a normal variant in that its origin is more posterior than usual and it enters the central sulcus above rather than at the level of the operculum.

On the right side, by comparison, there is a large posterior temporal artery that leaves the fissure proximally and two central sulcus arteries whose course and origins conform to the usual pattern. The internal carotid arteries on both sides (A, C) show the congenital coiling that may be held responsible for the stroke.

Although a field defect is usually associated with posterior temporal artery occlusions, it is not present in all cases.

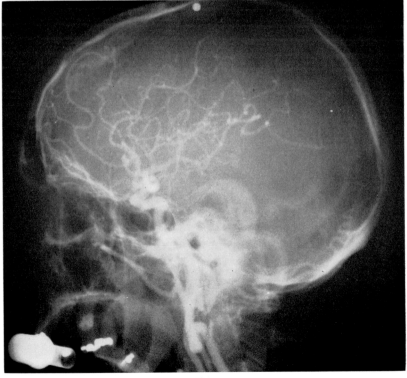

49A.

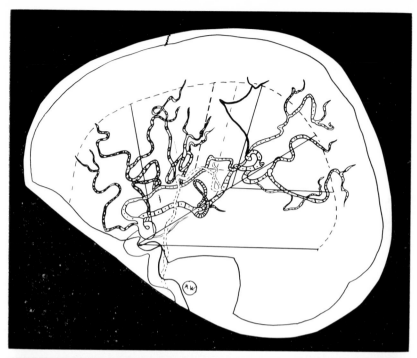

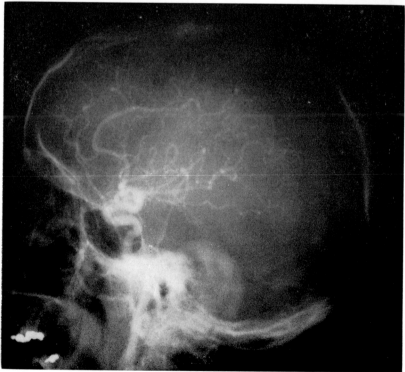

49B (*Upper*), 49C (*Lower*). See legend, page 163.

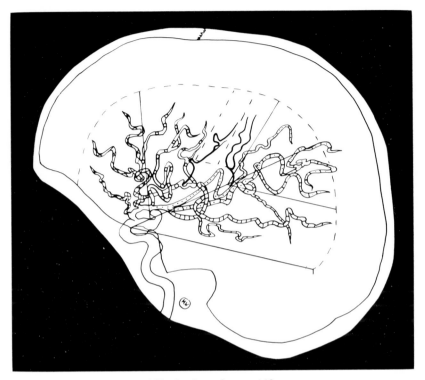

49D. See legend, page 163.

50. OCCLUSION OF ANTERIOR CEREBRAL ARTERY. AN INCIDENTAL FINDING?

This 70-year-old man had a stroke two years prior to admission with a residual right hemiparesis. His admission followed a second episode which resulted in continuous seizures involving the left arm and leg.

On the two frontal projections (A and B), a large anterior cerebral on the left is seen to end abruptly, filling part way from both right and left sides. Both pericallosal groups are supplied from the right and appear entirely normal. The old hemiparesis on the right might have been due to occlusion of Heubner's artery, but if one looks closely at the left lateral projection with drawing of the middle cerebral artery branches (C and D), the central sulcus artery is abnormally small suggesting an occlusion of one component or recanalization of a previous occlusion. On the right side (E and F), there are two large central sulcus arteries but the anterior component of the operculofrontal branch is extremely small similar to the central sulcus artery on the left.

It seems likely that the patient's seizures are due to ischemia of the premotor area on the right and that his hemiparesis was the result of a previous occlusion of central sulcus arteries on the left. While this is indeed microneuroradiology and may be disputed, it is difficult to explain the train of events on the obvious occlusive process in the left anterior cerebral artery.

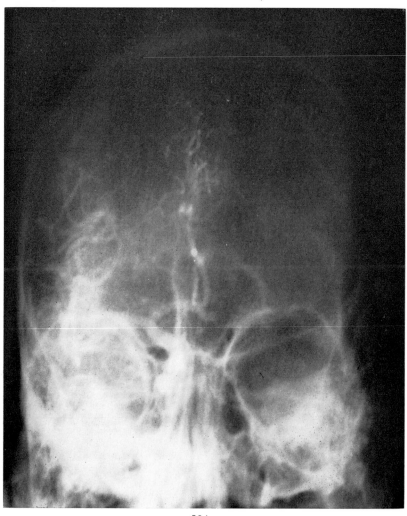

50A.

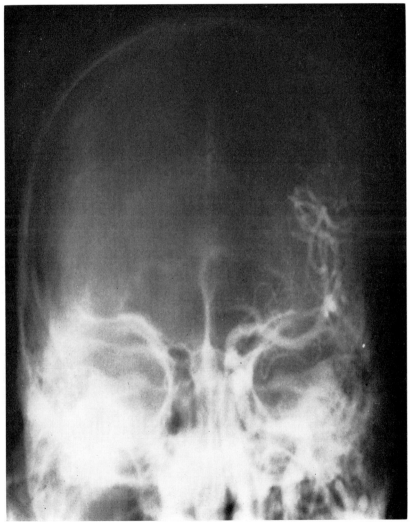

50B. See legend, page 166.

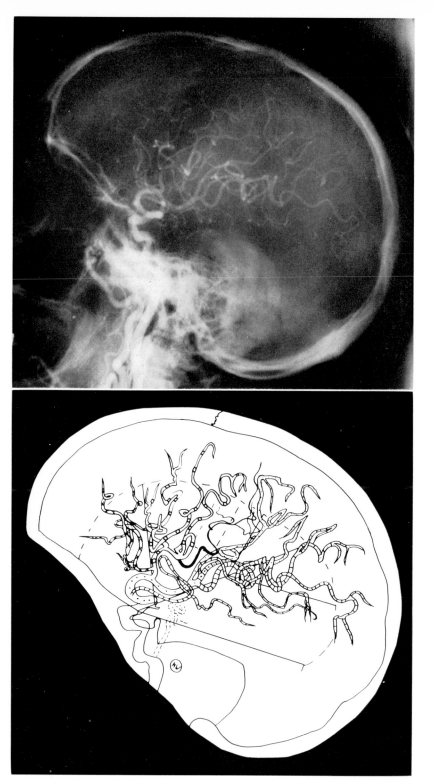

50C (*Upper*), 50D (*Lower*). See legend, page 166.

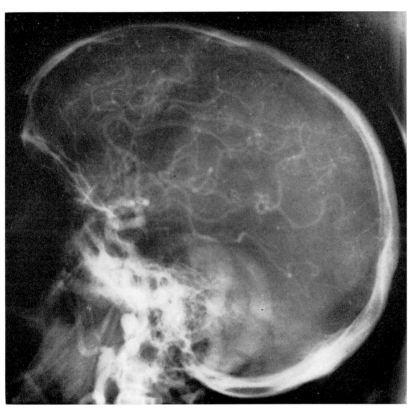

50E. See legend, page 166.

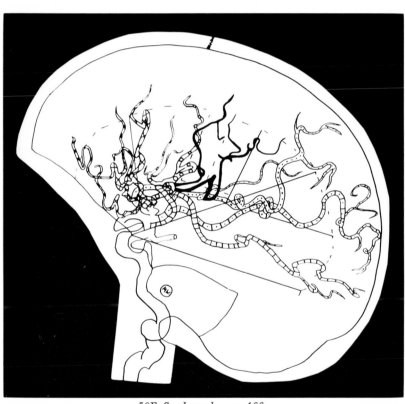

50F. See legend, page 166.

51. GROSS OCCLUSION OF PERICALLOSAL ARTERY WITH MINIMAL NEUROLOGICAL CHANGE

This middle aged man's illness was first manifest by an unusual and interesting complaint. He simply forgot to go to bed one night and was found by his wife in the morning in no distress and fully ambulatory but quite indifferent to his surroundings.

On the frontal projections both right and left (A and B), there is seen to be one large pericallosal artery that supplies the precuneus on both sides but is completely devoid of branches to the frontal lobe. On the lateral projection (C and D), the one pericallosal artery is equally well filled from either side and the branches of the ascending frontal complex are all unusually extensive, reaching high up on the convexity, better seen on the drawings (E and F). On later films, on the right there is retrograde filling of a pericallosal branch (G) and on the frontal projection (H) opacification of some branches in the region of the paracentral lobule is seen on the right side.

Unfortunately, it is impossible to be sure of the pre-existing anatomical arrangement. The only thing certain is that the arteries supplying the medial aspect of both frontal lobes are absent. Why retrograde collateral was only seen from the right side is not explained. It is even more difficult to equate the massive area devoid of vessels with the minimal neurological deficit but not only was this the case but the patient recovered almost completely and is again gainfully employed. The compensatory enlargement of the middle cerebral artery branches is probably related and there may have been a gradual stenosis as in the case with incomplete filling of the middle group, allowing the development of abundant collateral even though its radiographic manifestations is not prominent.

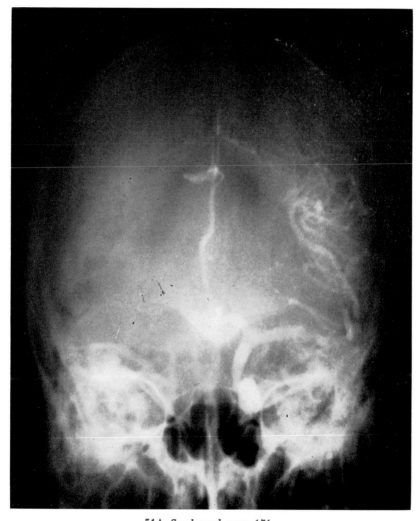

51A. See legend, page 171.

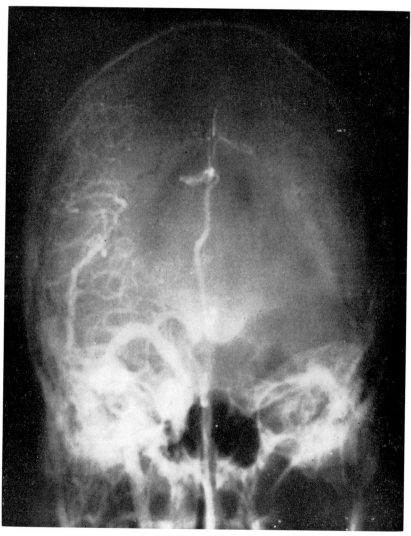

51B. See legend, page 171.

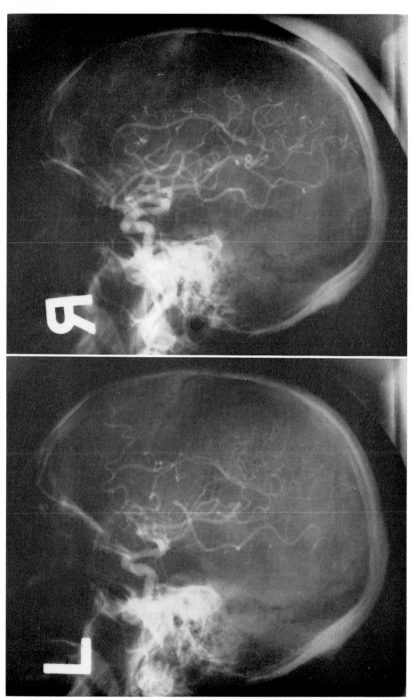

51C (*Upper*), 51D (*Lower*). See legend, page 171.

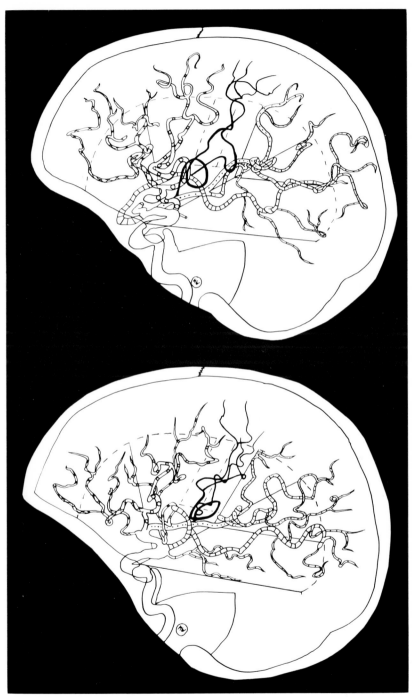

51E (*Upper*), 51F (*Lower*). See legend, page 171.

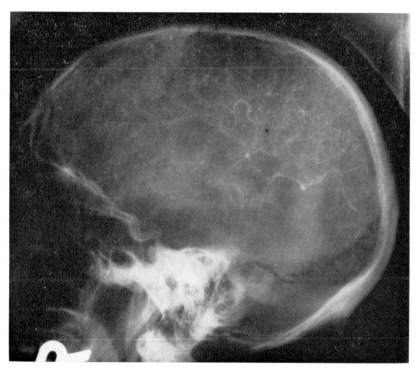

51G. See legend, page 171.

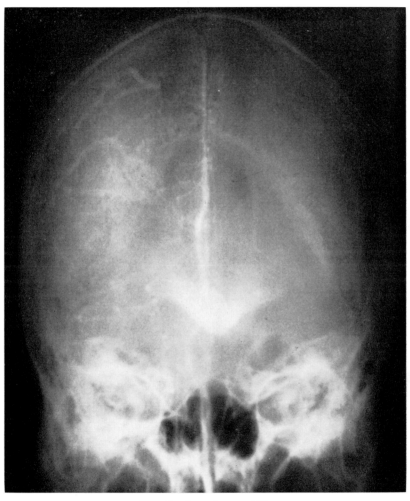

51H. See legend, page 171.

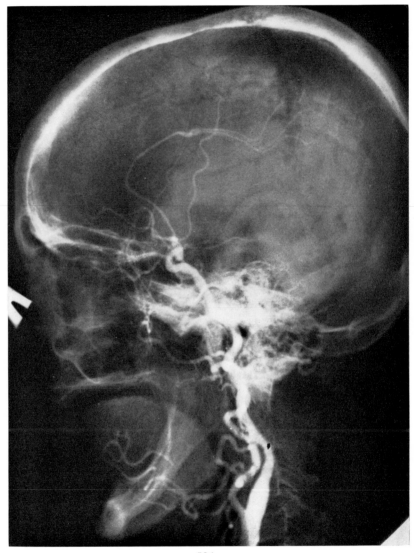

52A.

52. STROKE BEGETTING STROKE

When the brain herniates under the falx or in the tentorial notch, arteries may be occluded by pressure of the unyielding dural structures. The more abrupt the herniation the greater the likelihood of occlusion since the arteries have no time to adapt or imbed themselves in the softer brain tissue.

The lady above was an elderly nursing home patient, found unconscious on the floor and the angiogram done for fear of a subdural hematoma. There is complete absence of the middle cerebral artery, the pericallosal artery is

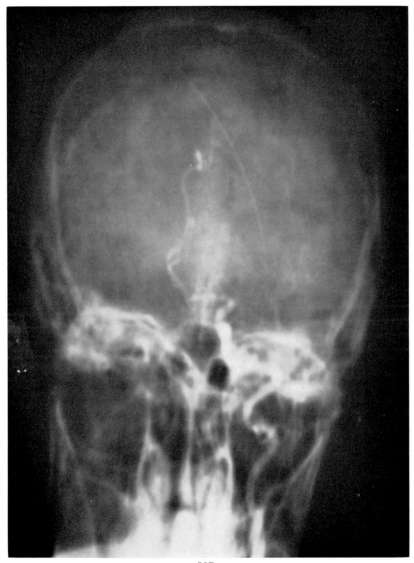

52B.

herniated under the falx and after giving off one good sized frontopolar branch has no further branching until reaching the posterior limits of the frontal lobe. Stumps of occluded vessels are seen on the frontal projection despite some blurring by motion of the patient. Burr holes on the affected side showed edema but no evidence of subdural hematoma. The edema in this case is presumed to be due to infarction. (Reprinted by courtesy of *Amer. J. Roentgenol., Rad. Ther. & Nucl. Med.*)

53. OCCLUSION OF POSTERIOR CEREBRAL ARTERY
DIAGNOSED BY RETROGRADE FILLING ON CAROTID ANGIOGRAM

This 48-year-old woman was examined for difficulty in vision. The neurological examination revealed only hemianopsia with macular sparing. On the carotid angiogram, the arterial phase is normal. There is a large pericallosal artery with abundant blood supply to the precuneus. The proximal portion of the posterior cerebral artery is faintly opacified.

In the venous phase, there is an arterial pattern posteriorly that does not correspond to any branches of the middle cerebral artery. The composite drawing of the middle cerebral branches to the area and the arterial branches filled by retrograde collateral prove that two different trunks are involved. The parieto-occipital and calcarine divisions of the occipital branch are especially prominent, the smaller branches running postero-inferiorly are probably terminations of the lateral branch, indicating that the entire posterio cerebral is occluded somewhere between the portion seen opacified on the carotid angiogram and the bifurcation into occipital and lateral branches.

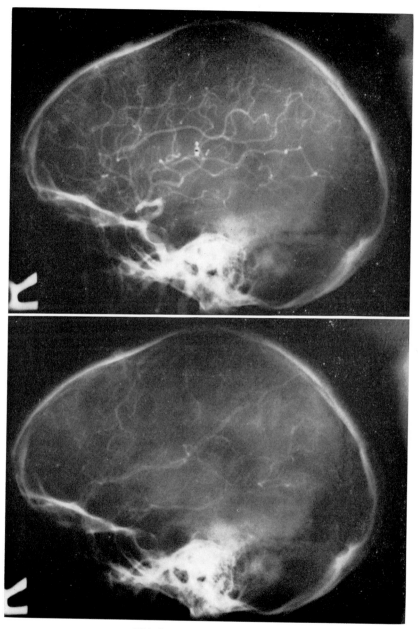

53A (*Upper*), 53B (*Lower*).
See legend, page 180.

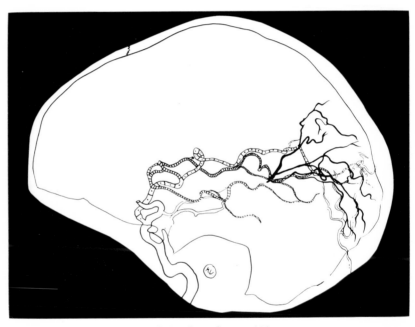

53C. See legend, page 180.

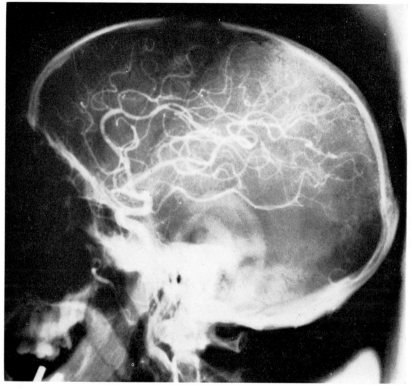

54A.

54. OCCLUSION OF LATERAL BRANCH OF POSTERIOR CEREBRAL ARTERY SEEN ON CAROTID ANGIOGRAM

This 50-year-old man was examined following a stroke that resulted in a visual field defect. There is elevation of the entire middle group (A) so that the posterior cerebral artery is seen with unusual clarity. There is complete absence of the lateral branch.

Drawing of the middle cerebral artery branches (B) shows the elevation of all vessels and the stretching of small branches from the posterior temporal that run down over the temporal lobe.

On the drawing of the pericallosal and posterior cerebral arteries, the calcarine branches are seen pushed upward and well above the expected position of the calcarine fissure while the branches in the parieto-occipital fissure, being medially situated, are normal in position.

The lateral branch of the posterior cerebral artery on rare occasions arises from the basilar artery as a separate trunk so that its non-filling on a carotid angiogram is not in itself diagnostic of an occlusion. In this case, the swelling of the temporal lobe in the area supplied by the lateral branch can best be explained by infarction and the clinical findings are confirmatory.

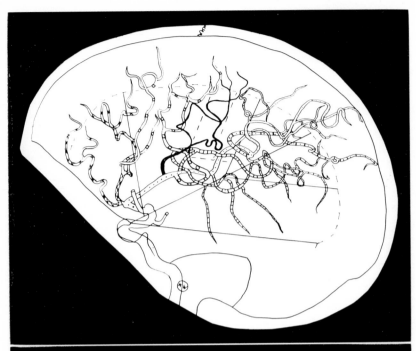

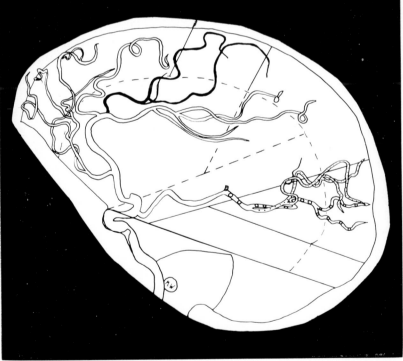

54B (*Upper*), 54C (*Lower*).

CONCLUSIONS

Before summarizing what we have intended to present, it may be fitting, as far as possible, to clarify any possible doubt as to what we have not intended to say.

First, we have not intended to infer that occlusive processes of the extracranial cerebral arteries are not important in the production of cerebrovascular disease. The numerous references to the over-emphasis on the role of the great vessels were made because, in our opinion, this has been over-emphasized, and over-emphasized to the point that other factors are being ignored. The theoretical likelihood of intracranial vascular degeneration occurring in association with lesions of the neck vessels; the frequency with which extracranial occlusions are incidental findings; the closer association of brain infarcts to arteriosclerosis of the intracranial rather than the extracranial vessels, and the discussion of concealed occlusions in which the carotid obstruction merely masks the actual disease-producing lesions, are intended to place stenoses of the neck vessels as a cause of cerebro-vascular disease in the proper perspective and not to ignore them.

Similarly, there is no intention of deprecating surgical treatment of extracranial occlusive processes. The only reservation implied is con-cern lest the enthusiasm for accepting extracranial stenoses as a major cause of cerebrovascular disease makes the indication for endarterectomy merely the presence of an accessible lesion. On the contrary, the frequency with which the carotid sinus has been the source of intracranial emboli in our experience suggests that surgical removal of the offending area should be endorsed with enthusiasm.

Newer modalities of investigation of cerebrovascular disease such

[185]

as the application of densiometric studies to cerebral angiograms, thermography, isotopic clearances or the Doppler effect using ultrasound to determine patency of vessels, are not discussed because they are not applicable to this particular approach to the problem and not because of any doubt as to their potential usefulness. Brain scanning has been only briefly mentioned for the same reason. However, in this respect, it is worth commenting on arguments as to the relative superiority of angiography versus brain scanning in the diagnosis of intracranial vascular disease. Such arguments seem similar to those of our medical predecessors when the auscultationist of the new school of Laennec battled those who favored percussion in the tradition of Auenbrugger, both sides proclaiming the value of their method and the disadvantages of their opponents. Angiography and brain scanning are not competitive but complementary, one reveals anatomy, the other pathological physiology. Brain scans reveal infarcts not detectable by angiography and angiography reveals a variety of vascular lesions, including occlusion that have not caused infarcts or infarcts not at the proper stage of evolution to concentrate the isotope, that are not detectable on scanning.

We do not intend to imply that all patients with evidence of occlusive cerebrovascular disease should be examined angiographically. Although in our experience direct carotid angiography is very well tolerated by the average stroke patient, this is not necessarily true under all circumstances. Patients with a generalized reduction in cerebral blood flow such as may be associated with border zone infarcts do not appear to tolerate the procedure as well as those with infarctions due to localized occlusions. The selection of patients for angiography remains a matter of clinical judgment and there is a standard expression among radiologists, probably based on the all too frequent sparcity of clinical information supplied with the request for a radiographic examination, that a good place to begin is with a history and physical.

In addition, it may be worth stating that this is neither a textbook of cerebral angiography or cerebrovascular disease but only a description of one aspect of both. Neither was there any intent of proclaiming the intracranial occlusions as the final answer to the problem. The limitations of angiographic diagnosis have, I hope, been dealt with in sufficient depth and fairness to give a factual and unbiased account of what can and what cannot be expected from cerebral angiography.

Having disposed of the negatives, it is much easier to state what has been intended. This is basically a presentation of anatomical facts applied to the angiographic diagnosis of a type of intracranial occlusion that in the past has seldom been recognized. Everything else is secondary and offered as supporting data. We believe this is important because the disease processes considered are common everyday occurrences that should not remain in obscurity. The potential for recognizing these small arterial occlusions exists in every institution where cerebral angiography is carried out and does not require vast expenditures for massive new equipment but only a little time and study by the individuals interested in the subject. It is hoped that the facts of anatomy presented here can ultimately be used for the benefit of the patient, if by no other means than by putting this aspect of cerebrovascular disease on a factual basis.

BIBLIOGRAPHY

ABRAMOWITZ, A.: See Romanul, F. C.

ADAMS, J. E.: See Newton, T. H.

ADAMS, R. D.: See Fisher, M.

AGNEW, C. H.: See Faris, A. A.

ALAJOUANINE, T., LHERMITTE, F., and GAUTIER, J. C.: Transient cerebral ischemia in atherosclerosis. *Neurology, 10*:906-914, 1960.

ALDERFER, H. H.: See Richardson, J. H.

ALLCOCK, J. M.: Occlusion of the middle cerebral artery: Serial angiography
as a guide to conservative therapy. *J. Neurosurg., 27*:4, 353-363, 1967.

ALMAN, R. W.: See Fazekas, J. F.

ALTER, M.: See Balow, J.; also Kieffer, S. A.

ALVAREZ, W.: Cerebral arteriosclerosis with commonly unrecognized apoplexies.
Geriatrics, 1:189-216, 1946.

ALVAREZ, W.: *Little Strokes*. J. B. Lippincott Co., Philadelphia, 1966.

ARING, C. D.: Vascular diseases of the nervous system. *Brain, 68*:28-55, 1945.

ARONSON, S.: See Soloway, H.

BAKER, H. L.: Medical and surgical care of stroke. Roentgenologic aspects.
Circulation, 32:559-562, 1965.

BALOW, J. ALTER, M., and RESCH, J. A.: Cerebral thromboembolism. A clinical appraisal of 100 cases. *Neurology, 16*:559-564, June 1966.

BANNISTER, R. G.: See Metz, H.

BAPTISTA, A. G.: Studies on arteries of brain. II. Anterior cerebral artery.
Some anatomic features and their clinical implication. *Neurology, 13*:825-
835, 1963.

BARNHART, M. I.: See Meyer, J. S.

BATES, B. F., and BOOKSTEIN, J. J.: Intercurrent embolization during cerebral
arteriography. Clinical and experimental observations. *Invest. Radiol., 1*:
107-112, March-April, 1966.

BAUER, R. B.: See Hass, W. K.

BAUM, S., STEIN, G. N., and KURODA, K. K.: Complications of "no arteriography." *Radiology, 86*:835-838, 1966.

BENDER, M. B.: See Mones, R. J.

[189]

BLADIN, P. F.: Radiologic and pathologic study of embolism of internal carotid-middle cerebral arterial axis. *Radiology, 82*:615-625, 1964.

BLOOM, S.: Pulmonary edema following a grand mal epileptic seizure. *Am. Rev. of Resp. Dis., 97*:292-294, February 1968.

BLUM, B., KOULI, N., LIBAN, E., and LEVY, P.: Paroxysms of T wave alterations in the ECG in experimental epilepsy due to foci in the pseudo-sylvian gyrus. Presented at the American Epilepsy Society Annual Meeting, November 1967.

BOOKSTEIN, J. J.: See Bates, B. F.

BOSCHENSTEIN, F. K.: See Wood, E. H.

BOSTICK, T.: See Edmonds-Seal, J.

BOSTROM, K., and GREITZ, T.: Kinking of the internal carotid artery. *Acta Rad. (Diagn.), 6*:105-112, 1967.

BRANDT, P.: See Tonnis, W.

BROADBENT, W. H.: *Clin. Soc. Trans., 8*:165, 1875 (quoted by Rob, 1960) *Proc. Royal Soc. Med., 53*:39, 1960.

BULL, J. W. D., MARSHALL, J., and SHAW, D. A.: Cerebral angiography in the diagnosis of the acute stroke. *The Lancet, 1*(7124):562-565, 1960.

BULL, J. W. D.: Use and limitations of angiography in the diagnosis of vascular lesions of the brain. *Neurology, 11*:2:80, 1961.

BULL, J. W. D.: See Metz, H.

BURNS, M. H.: See Fields, W. S.

BURROWS, E. H.: See Lascelles, R. G.

CHAIT, A.: See Gannon, W. E.

CHANG, C. H., and SMITH, C. A.: Postictal pulmonary edema. *Radiology,* 1087-1089, 1967.

CHASE, N. E., and KRICHEFF, I. I.: Cerebral angiography in the evaluation of patients with cerebrovascular disease. *Rad. Clin. No. Amer. 4*(1):131-144, 1966.

CHASE, N. E.: See Hass, W. K.

CHIARI, H.: Ueber das verhalten des teilungswinkels der carotis communis bei der endarteritis chronica deformans. *Verh. Dtsch. Path. Ges., 9*:326-330, 1905.

CHOI, S. S., and CRAMPTON, A.: Atherosclerosis of arteries of neck. *Arch. Path., 72*:379-385, 1961.

CHRISTOFF, N.: See Mones, R. J.

COLE, F. M., and YATES, P. O.: The occurrence and significance of intracerebral micro-aneurysms. *J. Path. Bact., 93*:393-411, 1967.

CONTORNI, L.: Vertebro-vertebral collateral circulation in obliteration of the subclavian artery at its origin. "Il circolo collaterale vertebro-vertebrale nella obliterazione dell'arterior subclavia alla sua origine." *Minerva Chir., 15*:268-271, 1960.

COOLEY, D. A.: See DeBakey, M. E.

CORDAY, E., ROTHENBERG, S. F., and PUTNAM, T. J.: Cerebral vascular insufficiency. An explanation of some types of localized cerebral encephalopathy. *Arch. Neurol. & Psychiat., 69*:551-570, 1953.

CORRELL, J. W.: See Wood, E. H.

COSTA, V.: See Montaldo, G.

CRAMPTON, A.: See Choi, S. S.

CRANDALL, P.: See Weidner, W.

CRAWFORD, E. S.: See DeBakey, M. E.

CRAWFORD, T.: Pathological effects of cerebral arteriography. *F. Neurol., Neurosurg. Psychiat., 19*:217-221, 1956.

CRITCHLEY, M.: Anterior cerebral artery and its syndromes. *Brain, 53*:120-165, 1930.

CONQVIST, S.: Total angiography in evaluation of cerebro-vascular disease: a correlative study of aorto-cervical and selective cerebral angiography. *Brit. J. Radiol., 39*:805-810, 1966.

CONQVIST, S.: See Laroche, F.

CROSS, J. N.: See Jennett, W. D.

DALAL, P. M., SHAH, P. M., SHETH, S. C., and DESHPANDE, C. K.: Cerebral embolism: Angiographic observations on spontaneous clot lysis. *Lancet, 1*: 61-64, 1965.

DALITH, F.: Calcification of the aortic knob: its relationship to the fifth and sixth embryonic aortic arches. *Radiology, 76*:213-222, 1961.

DALSGAARD-NIELSEN, T.: Some clinical experience in the treatment of cerebral apoplexy. *Acta Psychiat. Scand. Suppl., 108*:101, 1956.

DAVID, N. J., KLINTWORTH, G. K., FRIEBURG, S. J., and DILLON, M.: Fatal atheromatous cerebral embolism associated with bright plaques in the retinal arterioles. *Neurology, 13*:708-713, 1963.

DAVIS, D. O., RUMBAUGH, C. L., and GILSON, J. M.: The angiographic diagnosis of small vessel cerebral emboli. Presented at VIII Symposium Neuroradiologicum, Paris, September 1967.

DAVIS, D. O.: See Rumbaugh, C. L.

DAVISON, C., GOODHART, S. P., and NEEDLES, W.: Cerebral localization in cerebrovascular disease. *Arch. Neurol. & Psychiat., 30*:749-774, 1933.

DEBAKEY, M. E., CRAWFORD, E. S., COOLEY, D. A., and MORRIS, G. C.: Surgical considerations of occlusive disease of innominate, carotid, subclavian and vertebral arteries. *Ann. Surg., 149*:690-710, 1959.

DECKER, K. (Editor): *Clinical Neuroradiology.* McGraw-Hill Book Co., New York, 1966.

DELARUE, J., and GOUYGOU, C.: General etiopathogenetic data on atherosclerosis, considered from the anatomical point of view. *Rev. de L'atherosclerose, 2*:1-11, 1960.

DENNY-BROWN, D.: The treatment of recurrent cerebrovascular symptoms and the question of "vasospasm." *Med. Clin. No. Amer., 35*:1457-1474, 1951.

DENNY-BROWN, D., and MEYER, J. S.: The cerebral collateral circulation. 2. The production of cerebral infarction by ischemic anoxia and its reversibility in early stages. *Neurology, 7*:567-579, 1957,

DENNY-BROWN, D.: Recurrent cerebrovascular episodes. *A. M. A. Arch. Neurol., 2*:194-210, 1960.

DENNY-BROWN, D.: See Meyer, J. S.

DERICK, J. R., and SMITH, T.: Carotid kinking as a cause of cerebral insufficiency. *Circulation, 25*:849-853, 1962.

DERICK, J. R,. and SMITH, T.: Abstract—Carotid kinking as a cause of cerebral insufficiency. *Circulation, 25*:849-853, 1962. *Modern Medicine, 30*: September 17, 1962.

DEROUESNÉ, C.: See LHermitte, F.

DESHPANDE, C. K.: See Dalal, P. M.

DIAS, A.: See Moniz, E.

DILLON, M.: See David, N. J.

DuBOULAY, G.: Improvement in angiographic detail after hyperventilation. Presented in a discussion of the cerebral circulation. VIII Symposium Neuroradiologicum, Paris, September 1967.

DuBOULAY, G.: See Edmonds-Seal, J.

DUNBAR, H. S.: See McDowell, F. H.

DYRBYE, M.: See Gormsen, J.

EASTCOTT, H. H. G., PICKERING, G. W., and ROB, C. G.: Reconstruction of internal carotid artery. *Lancet, 2*:994-996, 1954.

ECKER, A.: *The Normal Cerebral Angiogram.* Thomas, Springfield, Illinois, 1951.

ECKER, A.: See Gensini, G. G.

EDDY, W. M.: See Ring, B. A.

EDMONDS-SEAL, J., DuBOULAY, G., and BOSTICK, T.: The effect of intermittent positive pressure ventilation upon cerebral angiography with special reference to the quality of the films, a preliminary communication. *Brit. J. Radiol., 40*:957-958, 1967.

EIKEN, M.: See Gormsen, J.

ENGELS, E. P.: The Roentgen appearances of carotid sinus calcification. *Radiology, 80*:436-437, 1963.

FALSETTI, H. L., and MOODY, R. A.: Electrocardiographic changes in head injuries. *Dis. Chest., 49*:420-424, 1966.

FARIS, A. A., POSER, C. M., WILMORE, D. W., and AGNEW, C. H.: Radiologic visualization of neck vessels in healthy men. *Neurology, 13*:386-396, 1963.

FAZEKAS, J. F., ALMAN, R. W., and SULLIVAN, J. F.: Prognostic uncertanties in cerebral vascular disease. *Ann. Int. Med., 58*:93-101, 1963.

FERRIS, E. J., GABRIELE, O. F., HIPONDA, F. A., and SHAPIRO, J. H.: Early venous filling in cranial angiography. *Radiology, 90*:553-557, March 1968.

FIELDS, W. S., NORTH, R. R., HASS, W. K., GALBRAITH, J. G., WYLIE, E. J., RATINOV, G., BURNS, M. H., MACDONALD, M. C., and MEYER, J. S. Joint study of extracranial arterial occlusion as a cause of stroke. *JAMA, 203* (11):153-158, March 11, 1968.

FIELDS, W. S.: See Hass, W. K.: see, also, Weibel, C. J.

FISCHER, E.: *Die Lageabweichungen der vorderen Hirnarterie im Gefassbild.* Zentralblatt für Neurochirurgie, Johan Ambrosius Barth, Leipzig, 1938.

FISHER, C. M.: Observation of the fundus oculi in transient monocular blindness. *Neurology, 9*:333-347, 1959.

FISHER, C. M., and KARNES, W. E.: Local embolism. *J. Neuropath. & Exper. Neurol., 24*:174-175, January 1965.

FISHER, C. M., GORE, I., OKABE, N., and WHITE, P. D.: Atherosclerosis of the carotid and vertebral arteries—extracranial and intracranial. *J. Neuropath. Exp. Med., 24*:455-476, 1965.

FISHER, M., and ADAMS, R. D.: Observations on brain embolism with special reference to the mechanism of hemorrhagic infarction. *J. Neuropath. Exp. Neurol., 10*:92-94, 1951.

FISHER, M.: Occlusion of the internal carotid artery. *Arch. Neurol. & Psychiat,. 65*:346-377, 1951.

FISHER, M.: Occlusion of the carotid arteries, further experiences. *Arch. Neurol. & Psychiat., 72*:187-204, 1954.

FOIX, C., et LEVY, M.: Les ramollissements syviens. *Rev. neurol., 1*(1927) 1.

FREDERICK, W.: See McDowell, F. H.

FRIEBURG, S. J.: See David, N. J.

GABRIELE, B.: See Ferris, E. J.

GALBRAITH, J. G.: See Fields, W. S.

GANNON, W. E., and CHAIT, A.: Occlusion of middle cerebral artery with recanalization. Am. J. Roentg. 88: 24-26, 1962.

GAUTIER, J. C.: Table rond sur la circulation cerebrale. Presented in discussion at VIII Symposium Neuroradiologicum, Paris, September 1967.

GAUTIER, J. C.: See Alajouanine, T.; also, LHermitte, F.

GENSINI, G. G., and ECKER, A.: Percutaneous aortocerebral angiography. *Radiology, 75*:885-893, 1960.

GILROY, J.: See Meyer, J. S.

GILSON, J. M.: See Davis, D. O.

GOFMAN, J. W.: See Young, W.

GOODHART, S. P.: See Davison, C.

GOODING, C. A.: See LeMay, M.

GORE, I.: See Fisher, C. M.

GORMSEN, J., DYRBYE, M., EIKEN, M., and RONNOV-JESSEN, V.: Acute cerebral infarct. Extracerebral genesis with particular reference to cardiovascular status. *Acta Med. Scand., 169*:455-466, 1961.

GOUYGOU, C.: See DeLarue, J.

GOWERS, W. R.: On a case of simultaneous embolism of central retinal and middle cerebral arteries. *Lancet, 2*:794, 1875.

GREITZ, T., and LINDGREN, E.: Cerebral angiography. In: Abrams: *Angiography,* Vol. 1, 1961.

GREITZ, T., and REUTER, S.: Methods of angiographic mapping of regional cerebral circulation. *Invest. Radiol., 1*:214-219, 1966.

GREITZ, T.: See Bostrom, K.

GRIFFITHS, J. O.: See Riggs, H. E.

GRUNDY, S. M.: See Jett, J. D.

GUIRAUD, B.: See LHermitte, F.

GUNNING, A. J., PICKERING, G. W., ROBB-SMITH, A. H. T., and RUSSELL, R. R.: Mural thrombosis of the subclavian artery with subsequent embolism in cervical rib. *Quart. J. Med., 33*:133-154, 1964.

GUNNING, A. J. PICKERING, G. W., ROBB-SMITH, A. H. T., and RUSSELL, R. R.: Mural thrombosis of the internal carotid artery and subsequent embolism. *Quart. J. Med., 33*:155-195, 1964.

GURDJIAN, E. S., HARDY, W. G., LINDNER, D. W., and THOMAS, L. M.: Analysis of occlusive diseases of the carotid artery and the stroke syndrome. *JAMA, 176*:194-204, 1961.

GURDJIAN, E. S., LINDNER, D. W., HARDY, W. G., and THOMAS, L. M.: "Completed stroke" due to occlusive cerebrovascular disease. *Neurology, 11*:724-733, 1961.

GURDJIAN, E. S.: See Webster, J. E.

GYORI, E.: See Winter, W. J.

HANAFEE, W.: See Weidner, W.

HARDESTY, W. H.: Minimum brain deficiency with occlusion of carotid and vertebral arteries bilaterally. *JAMA, 205*:7:527-528, 1968.

HARDIN, C. A.: The vertebral artery "pinch." *The Heart Bulletin, 15*:21-23, 1966.

HARDY, W. G.: See Gurdjian, E. S.; also, Webster, J. E.

HASS, W. K., FIELDS, W. S., NORTH, R. R., KRICHEFF, I. I., CHASE, N. E., and BAUER, R. B.: Joint study of extracranial arterial occlusion. *JAMA, 203* (11)159-166, March 11, 1968.

HASS, W. K.: See Fields, W. S.

HIPONA, F. A.: See Ferris, E. J.

HODES, P. J.: See Lee, F. K. See, also, Pendergrass, E. P.

HOLLENHORST, R. W.: Significance of bright plaques in the retinal arterioles. *Trans. Amer. Ophthal. Soc., 59*:252-273, 1961.

HOLLING, H. E.: See Reivich, M.

HOLT, J. F., and WHITEHOUSE, W. M.: *Year Book of Radiology,* 1959-1960 (p. 7-8). Year Book Publishers, Inc., Chicago, 1960.

HORTIER, W.: See Udvarhelyi, G.

Hsu, I., and Kistin, A. D.: Buckling of the great vessels, a clinical and angio-cardiographic study. *Arch. Int. Med.,* 98:712-719, 1956.

Huber, W.: See Welch, K.

Hultquist, G. T.: *Uber thrombose und embolie der arteria carotis.* Jena, Gustav Fischer Verlag., Stockholm, 1942.

Hunt, J. R.: Role of carotid arteries in causation of vascular lesions of the brain, with remarks on certain special features of the symptomatology. *Am. J. Med. Sci.,* 147:704-713, 1914.

Hutchinson, E. C., and Yates, P. O.: Carotico-vertebral stenosis. *Lancet,* 1:2-8, 1957.

Iannone, A.: See Zatz, L.

Ingersoll, C.: See Welch, K.

Irving, D. W.: See Corday, E.

Jennett, W. D., and Cross, J. N.: Influence of pregnancy and oral contra-ceptions on the incidence of strokes in women of childbearing age. *Lancet,* 1019-1023, May 13 1967.

Jett, J. D., and Grundy, S. M.: Studies on age and sex incidence of various diseases resulting from atherosclerosis. *J. Amer. Geriat, Soc.,* 8:245-256, 1960.

Johnson, J. F.: See Meyer, J. S.

Jorgensen, L., and Torvik, A.: Ischemic cerebrovascular disease in an autopsy series. *J. Neurolog. Sci.,* 3:490-509, 1966.

Jorgensen, L.: See Torvik, A.

Kaplan, H. A., and Ford, D. H.: *The Brain Vascular System.* Elsevier Publish-ing-Company, New York 1966.

Karnes, W. E.: See Fisher, C. M.

Katow, T.: See Nishimoto, A.

Keele, C. A.: Pathological changes in carotid sinus and their relation to hyper-tension. *Quart. J. Med.,* 2:213-220, 1933.

Kieffer, S. A., and Alter, M.: Serial angiographic evaluation of cerebrovascu-lar disease. Presented at VIII Symposium Neuroradiologicum, Paris, France, September 1967.

Kistin, A. D.: See Hsu, I.

Klintworth, G. K.: See David, N. J.

Koppang, K.: See Torkildsen, A.

Kouli, N.: See Blum, B.

Krayenbuhl, H., und Yarsargil, M.: *Die zerebrale Angiographie.* Georg Thieme Verlag, Stuttgart, 1965.

Krayenbuhl, H., und Yasargil, M.: Die angiogdiagnostische Bedeutung der Arterieae lenticulostriatae. *Neurochirurgia (Stuttgart),* 9:1-11, January 1966.

KRICHEFF, I. I.: See Chase, N. E.; also, Hass, W. K.

KURODA, K. K.: See Baum, S.

LANNER, L. O., and ROSENGREN, K.: Angiographic diagnosis of intracerebral vascular occlusions. *Acta Rad. (Diagn.), 2*:129-137, 1964.

LAROCHE, F., and CRONQVIST, S.: Angiography in cerebrovascular disorders. Presented at the VIII Symposium Neuroradiologicum, Paris, France, 1967.

LARSON, S. J., LOVE, L., and TIMMONS, C.: Segmental occlusion of middle cerebral artery. *Am. J. Roent., Rad. Ther. & Nucl. Med., 94*:223-229, 1965.

LASCELLES, R. G., and BURROWS, E. H.: Occlusion of middle cerebral artery. *Brain, 88*:85-96, 1965.

LEE, F. K., and HODES, P. J.: Intracranial ischemic lesions. *Rad. Clin. N. Amer., 5*:363-393, December 1967.

LEMAY, M., and GOODING, C. A.: The clinical significance of the azygous anterior cerebral artery. *Am. J. Roent., Rad. Ther. & Nucl. Med., 98*: 602-610, 1966.

LEVY, M.: See Foix, C.

LEVY, P.: See Blum, B.

LHERMITTE, F., GAUTIER, J. C., DEROUESNE, C., and GUIRAUD, B.: Ischemic accidents in the middle cerebral artery territory. A study of the causes in 122 cases. *Arch. Neurol., 19*:248-256, September 1968.

LHERMITTE, F.: See Alajouanine, T.

LIBAN, E.: See Blum, B.

LIMA, P.: *Cerebral angiography.* Oxford University Press, New York. 1950.

LIMA, A.: See Moniz, E.

LINDGREN, E.: Radiologic examination of the brain and spinal cord. *Act. Rad. Suppl.,* #151, 1957.

LINDGREN, E.: See Greitz, T.

LINDNER, D. W.: See Gurdjian, E. S.; also, Webster, J. E.

LOEB, C.: Strokes due to vertebro basilar disease. Quote from Loeb and Meyer, pp. 169. Thomas, Springfield, 1965.

LOVE, L.: See Larson, S. J.

LOWE, R. D.: Adaptation of the circle of Willis to occlusion of the carotid or vertebral artery: its implication in caroticovertebral stenosis. *Lancet, 1*: 395-398, 1962.

LUND, D.: Presenting a paper by RING, B. A. "Diagnosis of embolic occlusions of smaller branches of the intracerebral arteries." Amer. Roent. Ray Soc. Meeting, September 1965.

MACDONALD, M. C.: See Fields, W. S.

MALAMUD, N.: See Young, W.

MARSHALL, J.: See Bull, J. W. D.: see, also, Metz, H.

MARTIN, M. J., WHISNANT, J. P., and SAYRE, G. P.: Occlusive vascular disease in the extracranial cerebral circulation. *Arch. Neurol., 3*:530-538, 1960.

MARTIN, M. J.: See Whisnant, J. P.

MARX, F.: An arteriographic demonstration of collaterals between internal and external carotid arteries. *Acta Rad., 31*:155-160, 1949.

McCORMICK, W. F.: See Stein, B. M.

McDOWELL, F. H., SCHICK, R. W., FREDERICK, W., and DUNBAR, H. S.: An arteriographic study of cerebrovascular disease. *Arch. Neurol., 1*:435-442, 1959.

MEHREZ, I. O.: See Moran, J. M.

MERRITT, H. H.: *A Textbook of Neurology*, 3d Ed. Lea & Febiger, Philadelphia, 1963.

METZ, H., MURRAY-LESLIE, R. M., BANNISTER, R. G., BULL, J. W. D., and MARSHALL J.,: Kinking of the internal carotid artery in relation to cerebrovascular disease. *Lancet, 1*:424-426, 1961.

MEYER, J. S., and DENNY-BROWN, D.: The cerebral collateral circulation. *Neurol., 7*:447-458, 1957.

MEYER, J. S.: Ischemic cerebrovascular disease. (Stroke). Clinical investigation and management. *JAMA, 183*:237-240, 1963.

MEYER, J. S., GILROY, J., BARNHART, M. I., and JOHNSON, J. F.: Therapeutic thrombolysis in cerebral thromboembolism. Double blind evaluation of intravenous plasmin therapy in carotid and middle cerebral arterial occlusion. *Neurology, 13*:927-937, 1963.

MEYER, J. S.: See Denny-Brown, D.; also, Fields, W. S.

MILLER, J. E., VAN HEUVEN, W., and WARD, R.: Surgical correction of hypotropias associated with thyroid dysfunction. *Arch. Ophth., 74*:509-515, 1965.

MILLIKAN, C. H., SIEKERT, R. G., and SHICK, R. M.: Studies in cerebrovascular disease. V. The use of anticoagulant drugs in the treatment of intermittent insufficiency of the internal carotid system. *Proc. Staff Meet. Mayo Clin., 30*:578-586, 1955.

MILLIKAN, C. H.: The pathogenesis of transient focal cerebral ischemia. *Circulation, 32*:438-350, 1965.

MILLIKAN, C. H., SIEKERT, R. E., and WHISNANT, J. P.: *Cerebral Vascular Diseases.* Grune and Stratton, Inc., New York, 1965.

MILLIKAN, C. H.: (Editorial) Perplexities in cerebrovascular disease. *Ann. Int. Med., 58*:191-192, January 1963.

MITCHELL, J. R. A.: See Schwartz, C. J.

MONES, R. J., CHRISTOFF, N., and BENDER, M. B.: Posterior cerebral artery occlusion. A clinical and angiographic study. *Arch. Neurol., 5*:68-76, July 1961.

MONIZ, E., DIAS, A., and LIMA, A.: LaRadio-arteriographie et la topographie cranioencephalique. *J. de radiol., 12*:72-82, 1928.

MONIZ, E.: *Die cerebrale Arterographie und Phlebographie.* Handbuch der Neurologie. J. Springer, Berlin, 1940.

MONTALDO, G., and COSTA, V.: L'aterosclerosi del seno carotico. *Helvetica Med. Acta., 32*:642, 1960.

MOODY, R. A.: See Falsetti, H. L.

MOOSSY, J.: Cerebral infarcts and the lesions of intracranial and extracranial atherosclerosis. *Arch. Neurol., 14*:124-128, February, 1966.

MORAN, J. M., and MEHREZ, I. O.: Focal convulsions in carotid occlusive disease. *Arch. Surg., 93*:977-979, December, 1966.

MORRIS, G. C.: See DeBakey, M. E.

MOUNT, L. A., and TAVERAS, J. M.: A study of the collateral circulation of the brain following ligation of the internal carotid artery. *Tr. Am. Neurol. A., 78*:47-49, 1953.

MURPHEY, F., and SHILLITO, J.: Avoidance of false angiographic localization of the site of internal carotid occlusion. *J. Neurosurg., 16*:24-31, 1959.

MURRAY-LESLIE, R. M.: See Metz, H.

NEEDLES, W.: See Davison, C.

NEIRLING, D. A., WOLLSCHLAEGER, P., and WOLLSCHLAEGER, G.: Ascending pharyngeal-vertebral anastomosis. *Am. J. Roent. Rad. Ther. & Nucl. Med., 98*:599-601, 1966.

NETSKY, M. G.: See Sturgill, B. C.

NEWTON, T. H., ADAMS, J. E., and WYLIE, E. J.: Arteriography of cerebro-vascular occlusive disease. *N. E. J. Med., 270*:14-18, 1964.

NISHIMOTO, A., and KATOW, T.: A special type of cerebral vascular abnormality of the Japanese. VIII Symposium Neuroradiologicum, Paris, France, September 1967.

NORTH, R. R.: See Fields, W. S.; also, Hass, W. K.

OKAGE, N.: See Fisher, C. M.

PATEL, A. N.: See Toole, J. F.

PEABODY, G. L.: Relations between arterial disease and visceral changes. *Tr. A. Am. Physicians, 6*:154, 1891.

PEEL, T. L.: *The Neuroanatomical Basis for Clinical Neurology.* McGraw Hill Book Co., New York, 1954.

PENDERGRASS, E. P., HODES, P. J., and SCHAEFFER, J. P.: *The Head and Neck in Roentgen Diagnosis.* Vol. 2, 2d Ed. Thomas, Springfield, 1956.

PICKERING, G. W.: Transient cerebral paralysis in hypertension and in cerebral embolism. *JAMA, 137*:423-430, 1948.

PICKERING, G. W.: The question of cerebral angiospasm. Editorial. *Ann. Int. Med., 36*:1129-1135, 1952.

PICKERING, G. W.: See Eastcott, H. H. G.: See, also, Gunning, A. J.

POLLOCK, L.: Behavior and treatment of strokes in later life. *Med. Clin. North Amer., 40*:211-221, 1956.

POOL, J. L.: Cerebral vasospasm. *N. E. J. Med., 259*:1259-1264, 1958.

POSER, C. M.: See Faris, A. A.

POSER, C.: See Taveras, J.

PUTNAM, T. J.: See Corday, E.

RATINOV, G.: See Fields, W. S.

REID, J. D.: See Richardson, J. H.

REILLY, J. A.: See Wood, E. H.

REIVICH, M., HOLLING, H. E., ROBERTS, B., and TOOLE, J. F.: Reversal of blood flow through the vertebral artery and its effect on cerebral circulation. *N. E. J. Med., 265*:878-885, 1961.

RESCH, J. A.: See Balow, J.

REUTER, S.: See Greitz, T.

RICHARDS, P.: Pulmonary oedema and intracranial lesions. *Brit. M. J., 2*:83-86, 1963.

RICHARDSON, J. H., ALDERFER, H. H., and REID, J. D.: Response of eye and brain to micro-emboli. *Ann. Int. Med., 57*:1013-1017, 1962.

RIGGS, H. E., and GRIFFITHS, J. O.: Anomalies of the circle of Willis in persons with nervous and mental disorders. *Arch. Neurol. & Psychiat., 39*:1353-1354, 1938.

RIGGS, H. E.: See Wilson, G.

RING, B. A.: Middle cerebral artery: anatomical and radiographic study. *Acta Rad., 57*:4: 291-300, 1962.

RING, B. A.: Angiographic recognition of occlusions of isolated branches of the middle cerebral artery. *Am. J. Roent., Rad. Ther. & Nucl. Med., 89*:2: 391-397, 1963.

RING, B. A., and EDDY, W. M.: Calcification of carotid arteries. *JAMA, 184*: 866-869, 1963.

RING, B. A.: Diagnosis of embolic occlusions of smaller branches of the intracerebral arteries. *Am. J. Roent., Rad. Ther. & Nucl. Med., XCVI*:3:575-582, 1966.

RING, B. A., and WADDINGTON, M. M.: Angiographic identification of the motor strip. *J. Neurosurg., 26*:2:249-254, 1967.

RING, B. A., and WADDINGTON, M. M.: Ascending frontal branch of middle cerebral artery. *Acta Rad., 6*:209-220, 1967.

RING, B. A., and WADDINGTON, M. M.: Intraluminal diameters of the intracranial arteries. *Vasc. Surgery, 1*:3:137-151, 1967.

RING, B. A., and WADDINGTON, M. M.: The neglected cause of stroke: intracranial occlusion of the small arteries. *Radiology, 8*:5:924-929, 1967.

RING, B. A., and WADDINGTON, M. M.: Recognition of small artery intracranial occlusions. *Hospital Practice, 2*:11, November 1967.

RING, B. A., and WADDINGTON, M. M.: Occlusion of small intracranial arteries as a cause of stroke. *JAMA, 204*:303-305, July 29, 1968.

RING, B. A., and WADDINGTON, M. M.: Radiographic anatomy of the pericallosal arteries. *Am. J. Roent. Rad. Ther. & Nucl. Med., 104*:1:109-118, September 1968.

RING, B. A.: See Waddington, M. M.

ROB, C.: Surgical treatment of atherosclerosis. *Proc. Royal Soc. Med., 53*:38-40, 1960.

ROB, C.: See Eastcott, H. H. G.

ROBB-SMITH, A. H. T.: See Gunning, A. J.

ROBERTS, B.: See Reivich, M.

RODRIGUEZ, J. N.: See Stein, B. M.

ROMANUL, F. C., and ABRAMOWICZ, A: Changes in brain and pial vessels in arterial border zones. *Arch. Neurol., 11*:40-45, 1964.

RONNOV-JESSEN, V.: See Gormsen, J.

ROSENGREN, K.: See Lanner, L. O.

ROTHENBERG, S. F.: See Corday, E.

RUMBAUGH, C. L., DAVIS, D. O., and GILSON, J. M.: The fate of experimental autologous emboli. Presented at VIII Symposium Neuroradiologicum, Paris, September 1967.

RUMBAUGH, C. L.: See Davis, D. O.

RUPP, C.: See Wilson, G.

RUSSELL, R. R.: See Gunning, A. J.

SAFER, J. N.: See Wood, E. H.

SALTZMAN, G. F.: Angiographic demonstration of the posterior communicating and posterior cerebral arteries. 1. Normal angiography. *Acta Rad., 52*:1-20, 1959.

SALTZMAN, G. F.: Angiographic demonstration of the posterior communicating and posterior cerebral arteries. II. Pathologic angiography. *Acta Rad., 52*:114-122, 1959.

SALTZMAN, G. F.: Circulation through the anterior communicating artery studied by carotid angiography. *Acta Rad., 52*:194-208, 1959.

SAMUEL, K. C.: Atherosclerosis and occlusion of the internal carotid artery. *J. Path. and Bact., 71*:391-401, 1956.

SAYRE, G. P.: See Martin, M. J.; see, also, Whisnant, J. P.

SCHAEFFER, J. P.: See Pendergrass, E. P.

SCHICK, R. W.: See McDowell, F. H.

SCHWARTZ, C. J., and MITCHELL, J. R. A.: Atheroma of the carotid and vertebral arterial systems. *Brit. Med J., 2*(5259):1057-1063, 1961.

SELDINGER, S. I.: Catheter replacement of the needle in percutaneous arteriography. *Acta Rad., 39*:368-376, 1953.

SHAH, P. M.: See Dalal, P. M.

SHAW, D. A.: See Bull, J. W. D.

SHETH, S. C.: See Dalal, P. M.

SHICK, R. M.: See Millikan, C. H.

SHILLITO, J.: See Murphey, F.

SIEKERT, R. G.: See Millikan, C. H.

SMITH, C. A.: See Chang, C. H.

SMITH, T.: See Derick, J. R.

SOLOWAY, H., and ARONSON, S.: Atheromatous emboli to central nervous system. *Neurology, 11*:657-668, 1964.

STARR, M. A.: *Diseases of the Nervous System.* James T. Dougerty, New York, 1898.

STEBBENS, W. E.: Turbulence of blood flow. *Quart. J. Exp. Physiol. & Cog. Med. Sci., 44*:110-117, 1959.

STEIN, B. M., McCORMICK, W. F., RODRIGUEZ, J. N., and TAVERAS, J. M.: Radiography of atheromatous disease involving the extracranial arteries as seen at postmortem. *Acta Rad. (Diagn.), 1*:455-467, 1963.

STEIN, B. M.: See Svare, G. T.

STEIN, G. N.: See Baum, S.

STEPHENS, J. W.: See Welch, K.

STEVEN, J. L.: Some pitfalls in the angiographic diagnosis of intracranial tumour pathology. *Clin. Rad. (London), 12*:194-208, 1961.

STURGILL, B. C., and NETSKY, M. G.: Cerebral infarction by atheromatous emboli. *A. M. A. Arch. Path., 76*:189-196, 1963.

SULLIVAN, J. F.: See Fazekas, J. F.

SUNDT, T. M., JR.: See Waltz, A. G.

SVARE, G. T., TAVERAS, J. M., and STEIN, B. M.: Postmortem angiography of the cerebral vascular system. *Neurology, 14*:1149-1151, 1964.

SYMONDS, C.: The circle of Willis. *Brit. Med. J., 1*(4906):119-124, 1955.

TAKAYASU, M.: A case with peculiar changes of the central retinal vessels. *Trans. Act. Soc. Ophth. Jap., 12*:554, 1908.

TANDY, R.: See Young, W.

TAVERAS, J., and POSER, C.: Roentgenologic aspects of cerebral angiography in children. *Am. J. Roent., Rad. Ther. & Nucl. Med., 82*:371, 1959.

TAVERAS, J.: Angiographic observation in occlusive cerebrovascular disease. *Neurology, 11*:86-90, April, 1961.

TAVERAS, J., and WOOD, E. H.: *Diagnostic Neuroradiology.* Williams & Wilkins Co., Baltimore, 1964.

TAVERAS, J.: Progressive multiple intracranial arterial occlusions: A syndrome of children and young adults. Presented as the Caldwell Lecture, The American Roentgen Ray Society, October 1968.

TAVERAS, J.: See Mount, L. A.; also, Stein, B. M.; also, Svare, G. T.

THOMAS, L. M.: See Gurdjian, E. S.

THOMPSON, J. E.: Editorial. Cerebral protection during carotid endarterectomy. *JAMA, 202*:1046-1047, December 11, 1967.

TIMMONS, C.: See Larson, S. J.

TOMIYASU, U.: See Weidner, W.

TONNIS, W., BRANDT, P., and WALTER, W.: The roentgenological diagnosis of tumors of the corpus callosum with a contribution to the roentgenological anatomy of the anterior cerebral artery. *J. Neurosurg., 17*:183-196, 1960.

TOOLE, J. F., and PATEL, A. N.: *Cerebrovascular Disorders.* McGraw-Hill Book Co., New York 1967.

TOOLE, J. F.: See Reivich, M.

TORKILDSEN, A., and KOPPANG, K.: Notes on the collateral cerebral circulation as demonstrated by carotid angiography. *J. Neurosurg., 8*:269-278, 1951.

TORVIK, A., and JÖRGENSEN, L.: Thrombotic and embolic occlusions of the carotid arteries in an autopsy series. II: Cerebral lesions and clinical course. *J. Neurolog. Sci., 3*:410-433, 1966.

TORVIK, A.: See Jörgensen, L.

UDVARHELYI, G., HORTIER, W., and AZVIS, D.: Quantitative and qualitative evaluation of neuroradiological diagnostic. Procedures in 100 children below the age of 4. Presented at VIII Symposium Neuroradiologicum, Paris, September 1967.

VANDER EEECKEN, H.: Discussion of "collateral circulation of the brain." *Neurology, 11*(Pt. 2)16-19, 1961.

VAN HEUVEN, W.: See Miller, J. E.

WADDINGTON, M. M., and RING, B. A.: Syndromes of occlusions of middle cerebral artery branches. *Brain, 91*:4:685-696, 1968.

WADDINGTON, M. M.: See Ring, B. A.

WALTER, W.: See Tonnis, W.

WALTZ, A. G., and SUNDT, T. M., Jr.: The microvasculature and microcirculation of the cerebral cortex after arterial occlusion. *Brain, 90*:681-691, 1967.

WARD, R.: See Miller, J. E.

WATERS, E. S. G.: See Young, W.

WEBSTER, J. E., and GURDJIAN, E. S.: Observations on hemiplegia with middle cerebral artery trunk occlusions and with "normal" carotid angiograms. *Neurology, 8*:645-649, 1958.

WEBSTER, J. E., GUARDJIAN, E. S., LINDNER, D. W., and HARDY, W. G.: Proximal occlusion of the anterior cerebral artery. *A. M. A. Arch. Neurol., 2*: 19-26, January 1960.

WEIBEL, C. J., and FIELDS, W. S.: Tortuosity, coiling, and kinking of the internal carotid artery. II. Relationship of morphological variation to cerebrovascular insufficiency. *Neurology, 15*:462-468, 1965.

WEIDNER, W., HANAFEE, W., and MARKHAM, C. H.: Intracranial collateral circulation via leptomeningeal and rete mirabile anastomoses. *Neurology, 15*:39-45, January 1965.

WEIDNER, W., CRANDALL, P., HANAFEE, W., and TOMIYASU, U.: Collateral circulation in the posterior fossa via leptomeningeal anastomoses. *Am. J. Roent., Rad. Ther. & Nucl. Med., 95*:831-836, 1965.

WELCH, K., STEPHENS, J. W., HUBER, W., and INGERSOLL, C.: Collateral circulation following middle cerebral branch occlusion. *J. Neurosurg., 12*: 361-368, 1955.

WHISNANT, J. P., MARTIN, M. J., and SAYRE, G. P.: Atherosclerotic stenosis of cervical arteries. *Arch. Neurol., 5*:429-432, 1961.

WHISNANT, J. P.: See Martin, M. J.: also, Millikan, C. H.

WHITE, P. D.: See Fisher, C. M.

WHITEHOUSE, W. M.: See Holt, J. F.

WILLIS, T.: *The Anatomy of the Brain and Nerves.* Wm. Feindel, Ed. Tercentenary Edition. 2 vols. McGill University Press, 1966.

WILMORE, D. W.: See Faris, A. A.

WILSON, G., RUPP, C., RIGGS, H. E., and WILSON, W. W.: Factors influencing the development of cerebral vascular accidents. 1. Role of cardiocirculatory insufficiency. *JAMA, 145*:1227-1229, 1951.

WILSON, W. W.: See Wilson, G.

WINSOR, T.: *Peripheral Vascular Disease.* Thomas, Springfield, 1959.

WINTER, W. J., and GYORI, E.: Pathogenesis of small cerebral infarcts. *A. M. A. Arch. Path., 69*:224-234, 1960.

WOLLSCHLAEGER, G.: See Neirling, D. A.

WOLLSCHLAEGER, P.: See Neirling, D. A.

WOOD, E. H., CORRELL, J. W., and BOSCHENSTEIN, F. K.: Atheromatous ulceration in major neck vessels as a cause of cerebral embolism. Presented at VIII Symposium Neuroradiologicum, Paris, September 1967.

WOOD, E. H., CORRELL, J. W., REILLY, J. A., and SAFER, J. N.: Neuroradiologic evaluation of the results of surgical treatment of extracranial atherosclerotic disease. Presented at VIII Symposium Neuroradiologicum, Paris, September 1967.

WOOD, E. H.: See Taveras, J. M.

WYLIE, E. J.: See Fields, W. S.; also Newton, T. H.

YASARGIL, M.: See Krayenbuhl, H.

YATES, P. O.: See Cole, F. M.; also Hutchinson, E. C.

YOUNG, W., GOFMAN, J. W., TANDY, R., MALAMUD, N., and WATERS, E. S. G.: Quantitation of atherosclerosis. *Am. F. Cardiol., 6*:288-308, 1960.

ZATZ, L., and LANNONE, A.: Cerebral emboli complicating cerebral angiography. *Acta Rad., 5*:621-630, 1966.

ZAVIS, D.: See Udvarhelyi, G.

ZIMMERMAN, H. M.: Cerebral apoplexy; mechanism and differential diagnosis. *N. Y. State J. Med., 49*:2153-2157, 1949.

INDEX

A

Absence of intracranial branches
  as a congenital anomaly, 38
  as evidence of occlusion, 37
  in children, 39
Accessory
  blood supply to motor strip, 51
  parietal artery, 51-52
    illustration, 52
  temporal arteries, 53
Anastomoses, collateral circulation
    through, 10
  See also, Collateral circulation
Anatomy, normal
    illustrations of, 77-86
    intracranial arteries, 43-75
    post mortem correlation with
      angiograms, 77-79
Anemia, 31
Aneurysm
  aortic, as source of emboli, 107
  micro, 123
  spasm associated with, 13
Angiogram
  as crude procedure, 27
  correlation with brain scan, 158
Angiograms, normal
  due to lysis of embolus, 138
  with
    border zone infarcts, 138
    generalized arteriosclerosis, 138
    occlusion of penetrating arteries, 138
    transient ischemic attacks, 137
Angiography
  anesthesia in, 140, 141
  aorto-cervical and selective
    cerebral, 27
  four vessel, 15
  hazards of, 141
  hyperventilation in, 141
  limitations of, 137, 139
  normal in stroke patients, 137
  selection of patients, 186
  technique, 140-143

vertebral, anesthesia in, 142-143
  technique, 142-143
  vs. brain scans in infarcts, 186
Angular artery, 52-53
  occlusion of, 161-162
Anomaly, congenital, in absence of
  vessels, 38
Anticoagulant therapy, 12, 106
Anterior
  cerebral artery
    anatomy, 64
    horizontal limb, 64
    Lindgren's definition, 64
    occlusion of, 64, 65, 165, 166
    vertical limb, 64
  communicating artery, 65
  parietal artery, 52
  temporal artery, 45, 53
Aorta, emboli from, 107
  aneurysm, 107
Aortic
  aneurysm, 107
  arch study, 16
  knob, 4
Areas supplied by
  intracranial arteries, 43-75
    branches, 39
  middle cerebral artery branches, 57
    illustration, 74
  pericallosal artery branches, 67
  posterior cerebral artery branches,
    illustration, 74
Arteriosclerosis
  generalized intracranial,
    association with border zone
      infarcts, 136
    non-definitive diagnosis, 36
  of subcortical vessels, 139
  See also, Atherosclerosis
Aring, 13
Arteries, vertebral, pinching, 31
Arteritides, 32
Arteritis, 154, 155, 156
  "Japanese," 29

[205]